Maintaining a Healthy Lifestyle

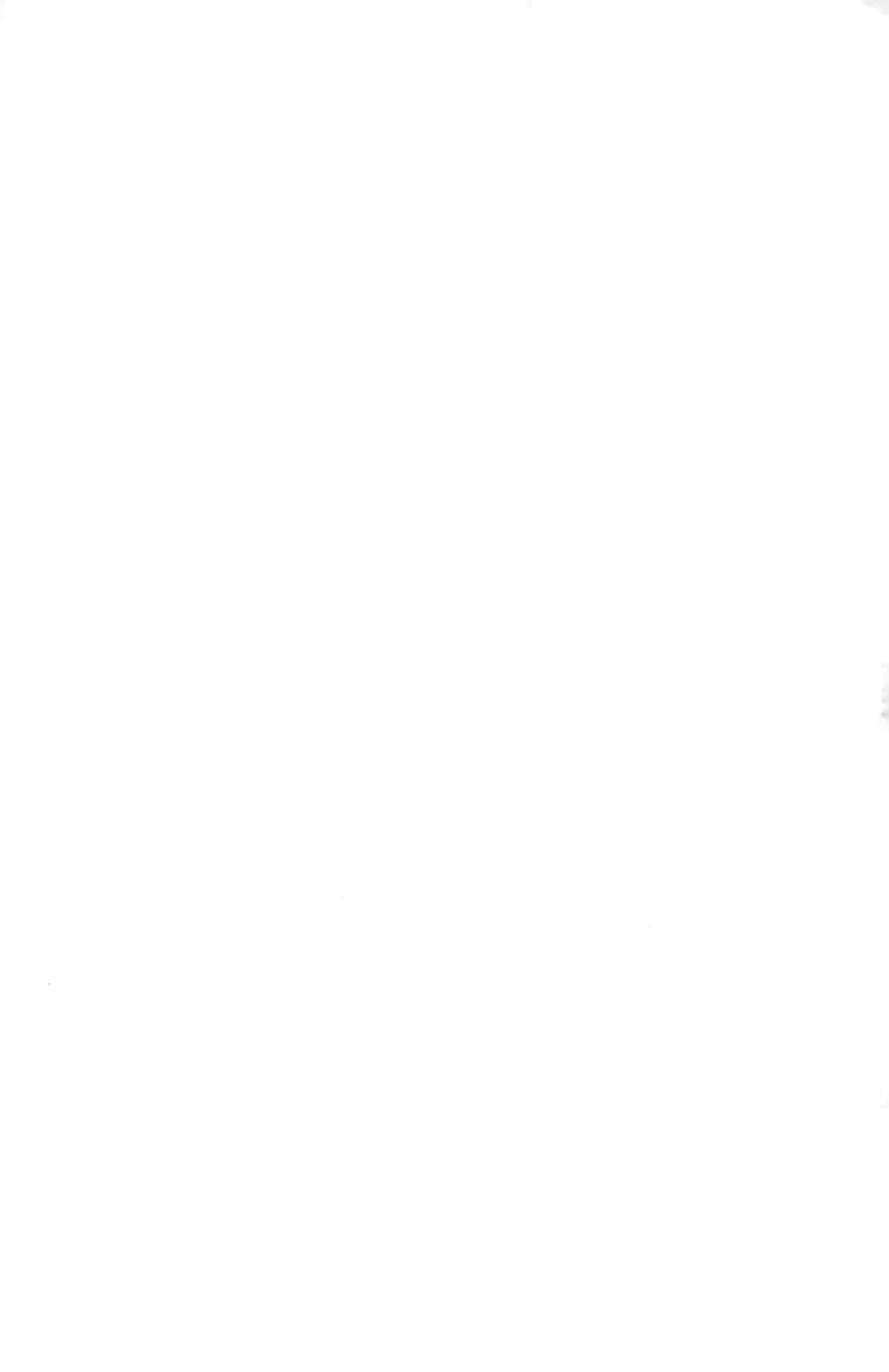

Adrienne Schäfer · Dorothea Schaffner ·
Karina von dem Berge · Nora Studer ·
Nico van der Heiden · Anja Zimmermann

Maintaining a Healthy Lifestyle

Psychological Interventions for the
Prevention of Chronic Diseases and the
Role of the Health Ecosystem

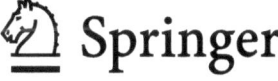

Springer

Adrienne Schäfer
Institute of Management and Regional
Economics IBR, Lucerne University of Applied
Sciences and Arts – School of Business
Lucerne, Switzerland

Karina von dem Berge
Institute of Management and Regional
Economics IBR, Lucerne University of Applied
Sciences and Arts – School of Business
Lucerne, Switzerland

Nico van der Heiden
Institute of Management and Regional
Economics IBR, Lucerne University of Applied
Sciences and Arts – School of Business
Lucerne, Switzerland

Dorothea Schaffner
Institute for Market Supply and Consumer
Decision-Making, University of Applied
Sciences and Arts Northwestern Switzerland
FHNW
Olten, Switzerland

Nora Studer
Institute for Market Supply and Consumer
Decision-Making, University of Applied
Sciences and Arts Northwestern Switzerland
FHNW
Olten, Switzerland

Anja Zimmermann
Institute of Management and Regional
Economics IBR, Lucerne University of Applied
Sciences and Arts – School of Business
Lucerne, Switzerland

ISBN 978-3-662-69459-6   ISBN 978-3-662-69460-2   (eBook)
https://doi.org/10.1007/978-3-662-69460-2

This book is a translation of the original German edition "Aufrechterhaltung eines gesunden Lebensstils" by Adrienne Schäfer et al., published by Springer-Verlag GmbH, DE in 2023. The translation was done with the help of an artificial intelligence machine translation tool. A subsequent human revision was done primarily in terms of content, so that the book will read stylistically differently from a conventional translation. Springer Nature works continuously to further the development of tools for the production of books and on the related technologies to support the authors.

Translation from the German language edition: "Aufrechterhaltung eines gesunden Lebensstils" by Adrienne Schäfer et al., © Der/die Herausgeber bzw. der/die Autor(en), exklusiv lizenziert an Springer-Verlag GmbH, DE, ein Teil von Springer Nature 2023. Published by Springer Berlin Heidelberg. All Rights Reserved.

This Springer imprint is published by the registered company Springer-Verlag GmbH, DE, part of Springer Nature.
The registered company address is: Heidelberger Platz 3, 14197 Berlin, Germany

If disposing of this product, please recycle the paper.

Acknowledgments

The present book contains the results of an Innosuisse research project. The research project was created in a collaboration between the Competence Center Service & Operations Management of the Lucerne University of Applied Sciences and Arts – School of Business, and the Institute for Market Offers and Consumer Decisions of the School of Applied Psychology of the University of Applied Sciences Northwestern Switzerland FHNW.

For almost three years, many other persons and institutions were involved in the project. We would particularly like to thank the representatives of the three business partners CSS, DR. BÄHLER DROPA AG, and uplyfe AG. In addition, numerous individuals agreed to participate in interviews during the various project phases. We would like to express our heartfelt thanks to them for the valuable insights into their respective professional and personal areas. Finally, we would like to mention Vanessa Feck and Julia Klammer, who actively participated in the project. We would like to extend our gratitude to them.

Contents

About the Authors

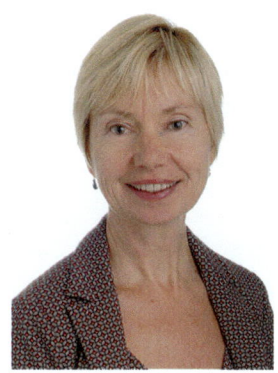

Prof. Dr. Adrienne Schäfer is a lecturer and project manager at the Lucerne University of Applied Sciences and Arts – School of Business with a focus on service management. She is the project manager of the research project "Sustainable Lifestyle Change".

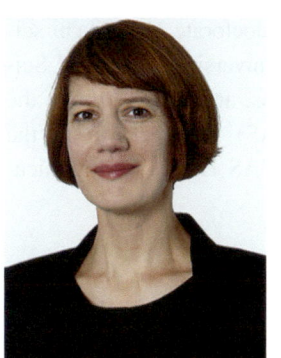

Prof. Dr. Dorothea Schaffner is a professor of economic psychology at the School of Applied Psychology of the University of Applied Sciences Northwestern Switzerland FHNW, with a focus on consumer behavior, interventions for behavior change, and sustainability. She is the co-project leader of the research project "Sustainable Lifestyle Change".

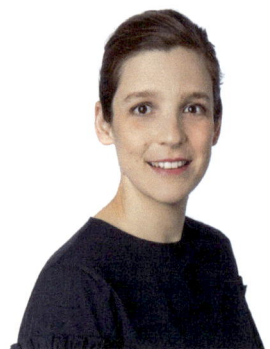

Karina von dem Berge is a Senior Scientific Associate at the Lucerne University of Applied Sciences and Arts – School of Business at the Competence Center Service and Operations Management and a doctoral candidate at the Cranfield School of Management.

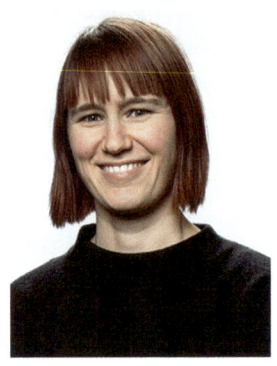

Nora Studer is a research associate at the University of Applied Psychology of the University of Applied Sciences Northwestern Switzerland FHNW. Her main focus is on consumer decisions and sustainability.

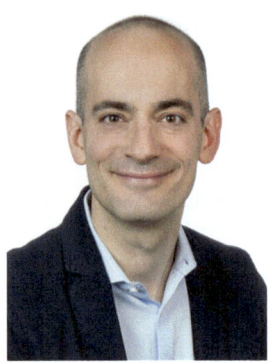

Dr. Nico van der Heiden holds a doctorate in political science, is a lecturer at the Lucerne University of Applied Sciences and Arts – School of Business, and co-director of the Master of Advanced Studies (MAS) Management in the Social and Health Sector and the CAS Health Communication.

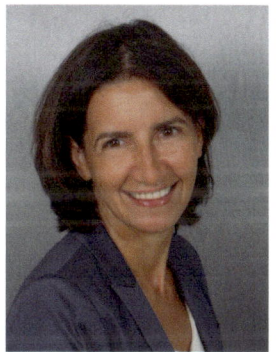

Prof. Anja Zimmermann is Head of the Competence Center for Service and Operations Management at the Lucerne University of Applied Sciences and Arts – School of Business, lecturer and program director of the Master of Advanced Studies (MAS) in Services Marketing and Management.

Part I

Introduction and Basics

Challenges of a Sustainable Lifestyle Change

1

Contents

Abstract

In Western societies, more and more people are suffering from overweight and are developing metabolic syndrome and/or type 2 diabetes. A sustainable lifestyle change, based on exercise and balanced nutrition, can prevent the onset of a disease, alleviate its course, or promote recovery. However, those affected find it difficult to sustainably change their lifestyle. Often, intervention programs are not aimed at sustainable behavior change and do not sufficiently take into account the motivational factors of individuals. As a result, those affected often revert to old patterns after some time. The applied research project "Lifestyle Change" deals with the question of how sticking to a healthy lifestyle can be supported from the perspective of motivational psychology and service management. This book focuses on the maintenance phase, which is central to the sustainable success of the lifestyle change.

© The Author(s), under exclusive license to Springer-Verlag GmbH, DE, part of Springer   3
Nature 2024
A. Schäfer et al., *Maintaining a Healthy Lifestyle*,
https://doi.org/10.1007/978-3-662-69460-2_1

1.1 Non-communicable Diseases—An Increasing Burden on Humanity and the Health System

Overweight and obesity (Adiposity) are increasing worldwide. According to the World Health Organization (WHO), 39 % of adults worldwide are overweight and 13 % are obese. Since 1975, obesity has almost tripled. Overweight is also increasingly a health risk for children and adolescents: In 2020, 39 million children under 5 years of age were affected, while among 5- to 19-year-olds, 340 million were overweight or obese (WHO, n. d.). Overweight is determined by the Body Mass Index (BMI). The BMI is calculated by dividing the weight (in kg) by the square of the body height (in meters). A person with a BMI value of more than 25 is considered overweight. If the BMI is above 30, it is referred to as obesity (adiposity) (CDC, 2021). According to the WHO, an increased BMI is an important risk factor for non-communicable diseases (NCD) such as cardiovascular diseases, diabetes, musculoskeletal diseases (arthritis), and some types of cancer.

Overweight and obesity often result from an energy imbalance between consumed and unused calories. This imbalance is promoted by an increased intake of foods that are high in fat and sugar. Furthermore, an increase in physical inactivity, for example due to the increasingly sedentary nature of many forms of work or the change in modes of transport (more motorized movement instead of muscle power), contributes to the energy imbalance (WHO, n. d.). Certain genetic predispositions and epigenetic changes also pose risk factors for the development of overweight and obesity (Fiedler et al., 2019). A diet rich in energy, fat, and sweet products and the resulting obesity often go hand in hand with massive physiological changes. Severe overweight leads to chronic inflammatory processes, which in turn cause epigenetic changes: The expression of responsible genes and the control of immune responses are permanently modified. It has been shown that although the inflammatory processes can be stopped by discontinuing the high-fat diet, the epigenetic changes remain and this can cause permanent, possibly lifelong changes in metabolic processes (Christ et al., 2018).

NCDs not only burden those affected and their environment, they also cause high costs for society. A distinction is made between direct and indirect costs. Direct costs are monetary expenditures made for medical and non-medical measures necessary for the treatment of the disease. Indirect costs do not involve money. However, there is a loss of resources, usually due to reduced productivity, e.g., due to absences from work. Intangible costs such as pain or grief are usually not taken into account in such cost-benefit considerations, as they are hardly quantifiable (OBSAN, n. d.; Wieser et al., 2014).

In Switzerland, 80 % of the direct health costs are caused by NCDs, similar to other Western countries. The treatment of the five most common NCDs (cardiovascular diseases, diabetes, cancer, respiratory diseases, and musculoskeletal diseases), which are often due to overweight and obesity, account for about 40 % of the direct health costs in Switzerland, annually over 25 billion francs (Wieser et al., 2014). Due to the usually long phases of illness, treatments for NCDs also last correspondingly long: They are care-intensive and thus cost-intensive. In the Swiss population, the five diseases mentioned above are also the most common causes of death (BAG, n.d.).

Overweight and obesity and the related NCDs, are largely preventable. According to estimates, more than half of NCDs can be prevented or at least delayed by a healthy lifestyle (BAG, 2016). The University of Halle-Wittenberg (Germany) was able to show with data from the international burden of disease study that in 2016, a million people in Europe died because they consumed too much salt, too many sugary drinks, and too many meals containing trans fatty acids (Meier et al., 2019). Research shows that in addition to the individual, the environment is also important in preventing NCDs. The environment is crucial in terms of how easy access is to healthy foods and regular physical activity. At the individual level, personal responsibility for a healthy lifestyle plays an important role. Responsible individuals limit their energy intake from fats and sugars and increase their consumption of fruits, vegetables, legumes, whole grains, and nuts. They also engage in regular physical activity. However, personal responsibility can only fully unfold its effect when people have access to a healthy lifestyle (WHO, n.d.). Accordingly, many government prevention and support measures aim to influence individual lifestyles and societal conditions (BAG, n.d.). The goal is not only to improve the health and quality of life of the population, but also to reduce the suffering of those affected and their relatives, as well as to save costs (BAG, 2016).

While many studies and government measures justifiably focus on the prevention phase, the question of sticking to a healthy lifestyle has so far been little researched. Many people who have once been on a diet are familiar with the so-called yo-yo effect. This refers to an unwanted and rapid weight gain after a reduction diet (Mühlemann, n. d.). It is known that the yo-yo effect can be reduced by regular exercise, and this is even more important than following strict dietary rules (Jakicic, 2008). However, this is precisely what many affected people struggle with. Therefore, the question arises: How can a change in eating and exercise habits be implemented in everyday life in the long term, without losing motivation after some time and falling back into old patterns?

National (e.g., NCD strategy in Switzerland) and supra- and international health promotion programs target the affected individuals, but also societal conditions. This fact is also taken into account in this book. Firstly, the individual and motivational psychological aspects of a sustainable lifestyle change are examined. Secondly, the perspective of Transformative Service Research (TSR) is adopted. Transformative service initiatives (TSI) refer to activities of public, private, non-profit organizations or volunteers. They advocate for people who are in a precarious situation and expect long-term problems with the aim of improving their well-being.

1.2   Psychological Perspective: The Challenge of Maintaining a Healthy Lifestyle

From a psychological perspective, the question of behavior change is central to a healthy lifestyle: How can the process of change towards a healthy lifestyle be described and explained? Psychological stage models, such as the Transtheoretical Model (Prochaska & Velicer, 1997), explain behavior change as a dynamic process along various stages: From the initial denial of the problem (e.g., weight gain is not perceived by the person affected as a health risk) to initial reflection, a wavering between "wanting to change" or "better not?", making a firm decision to change and the actual change, to the long-term maintenance and internalization of this behavior (e.g., going jogging three times a week and permanently implementing a diet reduced in fat and sugar). Ideally, the process of behavior change is undergone step by step. It is possible to discontinue the behavior change at any stage (e.g., I know it's unhealthy to eat sweets, but I still eat a piece of cake every evening). It is also possible for a person to regress and fall back into old and bad habits after a phase of healthy eating.

When it comes to change, the right timing is crucial. When accompanying and supporting those affected, it is important to recognize the stage of change, i.e., the phase of behavior change they are in. Each phase requires specific measures. For example, someone who has hardly thought about changing their lifestyle will be very reluctant to get involved in long discussions about their eating habits. A person who has already internalized a healthy lifestyle, on the other hand, will be interested in tips on how to maintain healthy eating habits over the Christmas period, for example.

This project focuses on the final phase of behavior change: in the maintenance phase, the aim is to establish and consolidate a new habit, i.e., a healthy lifestyle with sufficient exercise and appropriate nutrition. However, old behavior remains a temptation. People are faced with the challenge of resisting these temptations and dealing with setbacks (Prochaska & Velicer, 1997).

Behavior change is a process that each individual goes through differently. Based on the principles of positive psychology and the Self-Determination theory (Ryan & Deci, 2000; Seligman & Csikszentmihalyi, 2000), the present project postulates that those affected must develop an intrinsic motivation for sustainable behavior change, i.e., the motivation for a healthy diet and more exercise must come from the individuals themselves. With regard to the measures, this implies that they should also be aimed at intrinsic motivation in order to support the autonomy of those affected. To date, there have only been few scientific studies on health behavior with regard to these postulated relationships (see, for example, Donnachie et al., 2017). This book aims to contribute to closing these gaps in knowledge.

1.3   Transformative Service Research: Implementing the Service Orientation

Transformative Service Research (TSR) is concerned with services that "transform" the lives of service recipients. At its core, it examines the relationship between the service and well-being. TSR represents a relatively young and interdisciplinary branch of research that is aimed at solving complex societal problems (Rosenbaum et al., 2011). According to Anderson and Ostrom (2015), TSR addresses the well-being of individuals (micro level), service organizations (meso level), and industries or sectors (macro level), all three levels being interconnected (see Fig. 1.1). In the present project, the micro level refers to the affected individuals and their social environment, such as family members, friends. The meso level focuses on health service companies such as doctor's offices and pharmacies, and the macro level on the cantonal or national health system.

To better understand experiences at the individual level (micro level), the technique of Customer Journey Mapping is suitable. This refers to the structured and vivid representation of the experiences that a customer makes when purchasing a product or using a service (Lemon & Verhoef, 2016). The Customer Journey documents the experiences of customers during interactions with various actors, which can come from all three levels. If a person who wants to maintain a healthy lifestyle meets up with friends for a weekly running session, this is an interaction with another person at the micro level. If the same person goes for an annual check-up at a health center, they are interacting with a service provider at the meso level. There is often no direct interaction with actors assigned to the macro level, yet they have a decisive influence on the well-being of those affected. Examples include the cantonal and national health authorities, whose guidelines for product advertising for alcohol or cigarettes have a direct or indirect influence on the consumption of such products.

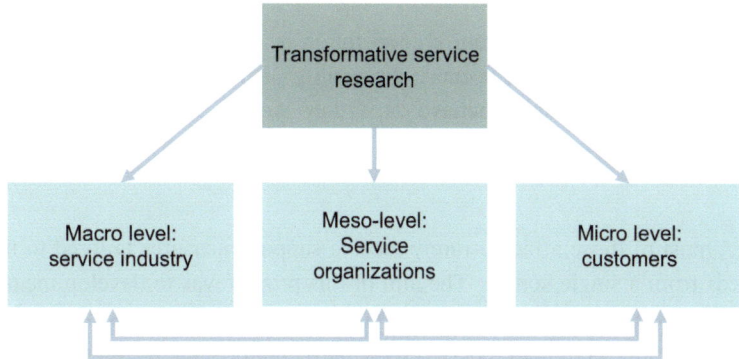

Fig. 1.1 Transformative Service Research in the health sector. (Based on Prentice et al., 2021, p. 2)

Services in general, as well as measures in the health sector in particular, are increasingly being offered in ecosystems in order to provide customers with a good or better service experience (Leimeister, 2020). The origin of the ecosystem view comes from biology. A natural ecosystem is a habitat in which different organisms coexist. To survive in this ecosystem, collaboration is often considered the most promising strategy (Farhadi, 2019). A forest, for example, consists of much more than just trees. In threatening situations, trees communicate with each other and protect each other. Underground fungal threads enable the necessary exchange, which in turn use the soil and the trees as a source of food (TED, 2016).

Moore (1993) transferred these mechanisms of action to the economy. Iansiti and Levien (2004) expanded Moore's approach and emphasized the independence of the individual actors. Although these individuals act autonomously, their individual success and ability to survive always depend on the other ecosystem partners. This in turn has a positive effect on the robustness of the entire ecosystem (Iansiti & Levien, 2004). The transfer of the ecosystem approach to the context of (service) management leads to a change in perspective from individual parts to the whole, from objects to relationships, from measuring to designing (mapping) as well as from structures to processes (Capra & Luisi,2014).

Similar to the natural phenomenon of trees, there are also many advantages for healthcare providers in offering services in a community:

1. Synergies in the transfer of knowledge and know-how can be realized.
2. Cooperations between independent providers means that risks and successes—in this case, giving up or maintaining a healthy lifestyle—can be better absorbed and distributed.
3. In a network, healthcare service providers can offer individual employees greater scope for individual development. In this way, they attract and retain talent in the long term (based on Farhadi, 2019).
4. Affected individuals benefit from a cooperation between the individuals and institutions providing the services, because the quality of health measures improves when providers in the community behave as if they were a single organism (Mancuso, 2018). The aim here is to offer support in maintaining a healthy lifestyle from a single source.

In practice, most of those affected rarely receive support measures tailored to their individual needs from a single source. The aim of this project was to develop measures that sustainably support the motivation of the individual affected and take into account the relationships and modes of action between the participants in the health ecosystem.

1.4   Research Questions and Approach

This book presents the results of an applied research project that focussed on the question of how affected people can be supported in sticking to a healthy lifestyle. There are gaps in knowledge about this so-called maintenance phase in research and practice, which this research project closes. It focussed on the following questions:

- What measures successfully support those affected in making a sustainable lifestyle change?
- What role do motivation and motivational orientation play in maintaining a healthy lifestyle?
- What does the maintenance stage look like and what customer journey do those affected go through?
- What role do those affected themselves and the other players in the health ecosystem play in a long-term lifestyle change?

The various questions were each worked on in interdisciplinary teams with researchers from behavioral psychology, health economics, and service marketing and management. The merging of different theoretical backgrounds, models, and methods, supplemented by various disciplinary findings and considerations, led to a holistic perspective of the project.

The applied research project was funded by Innosuisse, Swiss Agency for Innovation Promotion, and was conducted with three service providers from the healthcare sector (see Fig. 1.2):

CSS (https://www.css.ch) insures over 1.6 million people, making it one of Switzerland's leading health and non-life insurers. Its network consists of 100 agencies with 2700 employees. CSS stands by its customers as a health partner when it comes to staying healthy, becoming healthy, or living with an illness.

The Bern-based family business DR. BÄHLER DROPA (https://www.baehlerdropa.ch) maintains a network of drugstores and pharmacies at around 110 locations in German-speaking Switzerland. For over 50 years, DR. BÄHLER DROPA has been dedicated to the values of quality, commitment, and humanity in supplying people with medications as well as other health products and services.

Uplyfe (https://www.uplyfe.io) is a Swiss startup that uses artificial intelligence (AI) to support people with various nutrition and exercise programs to change and maintain a

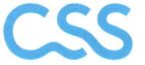
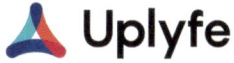

Fig. 1.2   The three practice partners

healthy lifestyle, relying on Artificial Intelligence (AI). Using a health app, Uplyfe offers personalized nutrition plans and also professional support on the path to a healthy lifestyle.

The research questions are answered in three steps, which are reflected in the structure of the book (see Fig. 1.3).

- The first part presents the basics. First, theories and applied research in health psychology are described (Chap. 2). Chapter 3 shows the basics and the current state of research from the perspective of service research and health economics.
- The second, empirical part presents five studies, combining qualitative and quantitative impact studies. In a first study, successful measures for sustainable lifestyle changes were identified through interviews with affected individuals and representatives from the health ecosystem (Chap. 4). A quantitative scenario experiment with 400 people affected was used to determine preferences for motivation-oriented measures and ecosystem touchpoints (Chap. 5). This experiment was supplemented by analysing the use of app data from Uplyfe (Chap. 6). A fourth study explored the customer experience of 20 people affected along the customer journey using in-depth

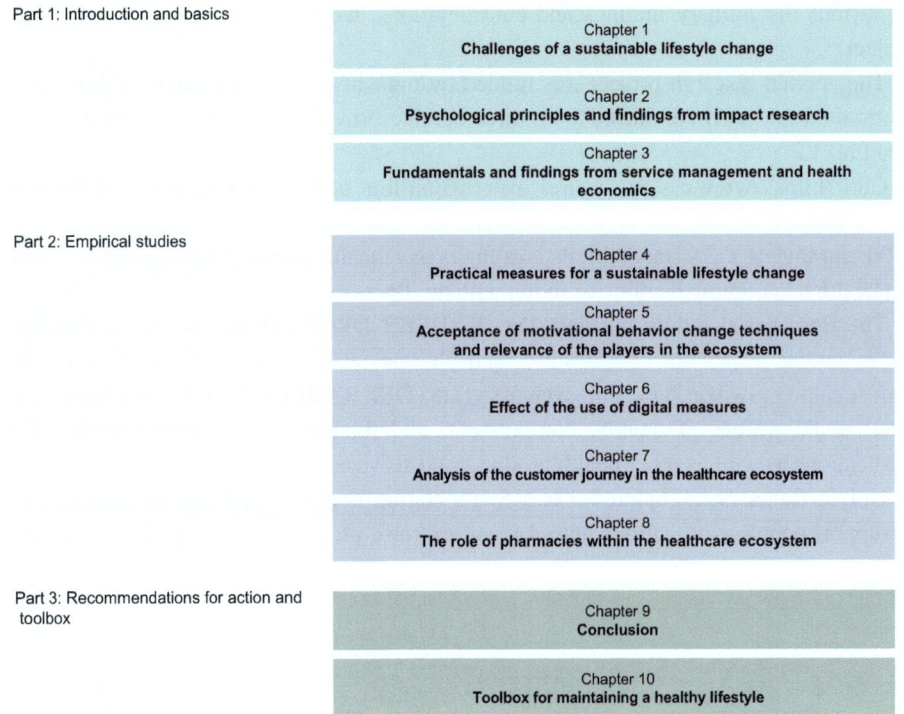

Fig. 1.3   Structure of the book

interviews (Chap. 7). Based on qualitative interviews with drugstore and pharmacy staff, a best-practice analysis was carried out as part of a fifth study (Chap. 8).

* The third part includes a conclusion and recommendations for action. The findings of the research project are summarised (Chap. 9) and the recommendations for action are presented in the form of a toolbox (Chap. 10). They are used to develop services to support those affected in sustainably changing their behavior during the maintenance phase. This will contribute to the prevention of non-communicable diseases and improve the chances of recovery. At the same time, the findings serve to further develop a health ecosystem that effectively and efficiently supports those affected in maintaining a healthy lifestyle.

References

Anderson, L., & Ostrom, A. L. (2015). Transformative service research: Advancing our knowledge about service and well-being. *Journal of Service Research,18*(3), 243–249. https://doi.org/10.1177/1094670515591316.

BAG. (n. d.). Nationale Strategie zur Prävention nichtübertragbarer Krankheiten. https://www.bag.admin.ch/bag/de/home/strategie-und-politik/nationale-gesundheitsstrategien/strategie-nicht-uebertragbare-krankheiten.html. Accessed 18. Oct. 2021.

BAG. (2016). Faktenblatt Nichtübertragbare Krankheiten (NCD). https://www.bag.admin.ch/bag/de/home/strategie-und-politik/nationale-gesundheitsstrategien/strategie-nicht-uebertragbare-krankheiten.html.

Capra, F., & Luisi, P. L. (2014). *The systems view of life: A unifying vision.* Cambridge University Press.

CDC. (2021). Defining adult overweight and obesity. *Centers for disease control and prevention.* https://www.cdc.gov/obesity/adult/defining.html.

Christ, A., Günther, P., Lauterbach, M. A. R., Duewell, P., Biswas, D., Pelka, K., Scholz, C. J., Oosting, M., Haendler, K., Baßler, K., Klee, K., Schulte-, J., Ulas, T., Moorlag, S. J. C. F. M., Kumar, V., Park, M. H., Joosten, L. A. B., Groh, L. A., Riksen, N. P., & Latz, E. (2018). Western diet triggers NLRP3-dependent innate immune reprogramming. *Cell,172*(1–2), 162–175. https://doi.org/10.1016/j.cell.2017.12.013.

Donnachie, C., Wyke, S., Mutrie, N., & Hunt, K. (2017). 'It's like a personal motivator that you carried around wi' you': Utilising self-determination theory to understand men's experiences of using pedometers to increase physical activity in a weight management programme. *International Journal of Behavioral Nutrition and Physical Activity,14*(1), 1–14. https://doi.org/10.1186/s12966-017-0505-z.

Farhadi, N. (Ed.). (2019). *Grundlagen: Gemeinsam stärker sein. Cross-Industry Ecosystems: Grundlagen,Archetypen,Modelle und strategische Ansätze* (S. 5–22). Springer Fachmedien. https://doi.org/10.1007/978-3-658-26129-0_2.

Fiedler, K., Hauner, H., Hertwig, R., Huber, G., Mata, J., Rösler, F., Roosen, J., Stroebe, W., & von Braun, J. (2019). *Übergewicht und Adipositas:Thesen und Empfehlungen zur Eindämmung der Epidemie.* Deutsche Akademie der Naturforscher Leopoldina e. V.—Nationale Akademie der Wissenschaften.

Iansiti, M., & Levien, R. (2004). Strategy as ecology. *Harvard Business Review, 82*(3), 68–78, 126.

Jakicic, J. M. (2008). Effect of exercise on 24-month weight loss maintenance in overweight women. *Archives of Internal Medicine,168*(14), 1550. https://doi.org/10.1001/archinte.168.14.1550.

Leimeister, J. M. (2020). *Dienstleistungsengineering und -management: Data-driven service innovation* (2. Aufl.). Springer Gabler. https://doi.org/10.1007/978-3-662-59858-0.

Lemon, K. N., & Verhoef, P. C. (2016). Understanding customer experience throughout the customer journey. *Journal of Marketing,80*(6), 69–96. https://doi.org/10.1509/jm.15.0420.

Mancuso, S. (2018). *The revolutionary genius of plants: A new understanding of plant intelligence and behavior.* Blackstone Pub.

Meier, T., Gräfe, K., Senn, F., Sur, P., Stangl, G. I., Dawczynski, C., März, W., Kleber, M. E., & Lorkowski, S. (2019). Cardiovascular mortality attributable to dietary risk factors in 51 countries in the WHO European region from 1990 to 2016: A systematic analysis of the global burden of disease study. *European Journal of Epidemiology,34*(1), 37–55. https://doi.org/10.1007/s10654-018-0473-x.

Moore, J. F. (1993). Predators and prey: A new ecology of competition. *Harvard Business Review.* https://hbr.org/1993/05/predators-and-prey-a-new-ecology-of-competition.

Mühlemann, P. (n. d.). Jojo-Effekt. https://www.feel-ok.ch/de_CH/jugendliche/themen/ich_und_mein_gewicht/rund_ums_thema_koerpergewicht/diaeten/diaeten/jojo-effekt.cfm. Accessed 7. March 2022.

OBSAN. (n. d.). Volkswirtschaftliche Kosten von NCDs. https://www.obsan.admin.ch/de/indikatoren/MonAM/volkswirtschaftliche-kosten-von-ncds. Accessed 18. Oct. 2021.

Prentice, C., Altinay, L., & Woodside, A. G. (2021). Transformative service research and COVID-19. *The Service Industries Journal,41*(1–2), 1–8. https://doi.org/10.1080/02642069.2021.1883262.

Prochaska, J. O., & Velicer, W. F. (1997). The transtheoretical change. *The Science of Health Promotion,12*(1), 38–48.

Rosenbaum, M., Corus, C., Ostrom, A., Anderson, L., Fisk, R., Gallan, A., Giraldo, M., Mende, M., Mulder, M., Rayburn, S., Shirahada, K., & Williams, J. (2011). *Conceptualisation and aspirations of transformative service research* (SSRN Scholarly Paper ID 2643219). Social Science Research Network. https://papers.ssrn.com/abstract=2643219.

Ryan, R. M., & Deci, E. L. (2000). Self-determination theory and the facilitation of intrinsic motivation, social development, and well-being. *American Psychologist,55*(1), 68–78. https://doi.org/10.1037/0003-066X.55.1.68.

Seligman, M. E. P., & Csikszentmihalyi, M. (2000). Positive psychology: An introduction. *American Psychologist,55*(1), 5–14. https://doi.org/10.1037/0003-066X.55.1.5.

TED. (2016, August 30). How trees talk to each other | Suzanne Simard. https://www.youtube.com/watch?v=Un2yBgIAxYs.

WHO. (n. d.). Obesity and overweight. https://www.who.int/news-room/fact-sheets/detail/obesity-and-overweight. Accessed 11. Oct. 2021.

Wieser, S., Tomonaga, Y., Riguzzi, M., Fischer, B., Telser, H., Pletscher, M., Eichler, K., Trost, M., & Schwenkglenks, M. (2014). *Die Kosten der nichtübertragbaren Krankheiten in der Schweiz: Schlussbericht.* https://doi.org/10.5167/UZH-103453.

Psychological Foundations and Insights from Research on Effectiveness

Contents

Abstract

Behavioral changes are a complex interplay of cognitive and emotional processes. The stage models of behavior change describe the different stages of this process. According to the Transtheoretical Model, behavior change consists of five stages: 1) Precontemplation, 2) Contemplation, 3) Preparation, 4) Action, and 5) Maintenance. The COM-B model describes that capability, opportunity, and motivation together can explain a behavior. Processes that regulate behavior can be influenced with behavior change techniques. In addition, the type of motivation and self-management play an important role in relation to a sustainable lifestyle change.

A. Schäfer et al., *Maintaining a Healthy Lifestyle*,
https://doi.org/10.1007/978-3-662-69460-2_2

Psychological processes play a central role in the behavioral change towards a healthy lifestyle. This chapter is dedicated to the relevant background from social and health psychology. First, the origins of psychological research on behavioral change are presented. The focus is on stage models of behavior change. After an explanation of general models, a deep dive into models from health psychology follows. Subsequently, the state of research on interventions for behavior change is presented. Intervention is the comprehensive collective term for all actions planned and implemented in the context of a behavioral change. Central is the concept of behavior change technique as a clearly distinguishable part of an intervention, which supports the behavioral change. The concrete implementation of a behavior change technique is then referred to as a measure. The chapter provides a classification of behavior change techniques and gives an overview of the state of research on their effectiveness. Finally, there is a discussion of the psychological foundations of motivation and self-management and relates these to lifestyle change.

2.1   Models of Behavior Change

From the early beginnings of scientific behavioral research and psychology, researchers have been concerned with the question of behavior change. Two similar approaches dominated the discussion (Bamberg, 2012): *firstly*, the economic approach of rational choice theory. Based on the image of humans as "Homo Oeconomicus", people make decisions based on rational arguments and change their behavior due to a logical weighing of the pros and cons of a behavior. Many behavioral change programs still assume today, based on this approach, that comprehensive information about the benefits of a healthy lifestyle can achieve behavioral change. However, later research from descriptive decision theory (e.g., Tversky & Kahneman, 1974) was able to empirically demonstrate that rational choice theory falls short and can only partially explain actual behavior. Therefore, other factors must be considered in explaining behavioral change.

Secondly, behaviorism provided an important basis for explaining behavior or behavior changes. The concept of human nature underlying this approach sees people as passive organisms that can be controlled by simple and short-term principles of pleasure gain and thus by reward and punishment.

Both the economic decision theory and behaviorism do not take into account more complex cognitive processes of motivation and goal orientation. These shortcomings in explaining behavioral changes are addressed in more modern theories of behavior change and self-regulation. These theories postulate that not only rational arguments, e.g., about pros and cons or short-term reward or punishment, can explain behavior, but internal processes of motivation, emotions, values, and goal setting are of central importance. These self-regulation theories are based on a concept of human nature that grants individuals the ability to set self-directed goals and invest time and resources in their achievement (Bamberg, 2012). Based on these approaches, behavioral change is a complex process involving an interplay of cognitive and emotional processes. The two most relevant approaches for the present study are presented below: the stage models of behavioral change and the COM-B model. The stage model describes behavioral change as a process with several stages, while the COM-B model identifies influencing factors on behavioral change.

2.1.1 Stage Models of Behavioral Change

One of the first theories defining behavioral change as a process is Lewin's stage model of change (1951). This simple model describes that individuals and groups go through three stages during behavior changes (see Fig. 2.1). In the stage of unfreeze, old behaviors are discarded and motivation for new behavior is developed. The stage of change is characterized by trying out and testing new behaviors. In the last stage, the refreezing stage, the new behavior becomes a habit.

According to this approach, the motivation to change arises from a perceived discrepancy between the current state (e.g., a person is overweight) and a person's goal (e.g., to be a healthy person).

Stage models of self-regulation are widely used in health psychology. The aspect of motivation is integrated as a central element in the more modern theories of self-regulation. Behavioral change is driven by the complex interplay of cognitive and emotional processes in which individuals compare their goals with the current state and negative emotions are triggered in case of a discrepancy.

Another central aspect of self-regulation theories is the temporal dimension: behavioral change takes time. In addition, the process of behavior change does not proceed uniformly, but—as already outlined in Lewin's model—stages are distinguished. Changes are always accompanied by feedback loops. It is important to note that the process is not completed with the last stage, but leads back to the first stage of behavioral change.

One of the most well-known stage models is the Transtheoretical Model of Behavior Change (Prochaska & Velicer, 1997). The Transtheoretical Model is a comprehensive model for explaining and designing behavior changes. It builds on the basic ideas of Lewin and further differentiates the stages of behavior change. The model distinguishes

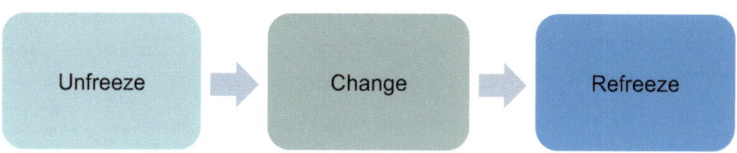

Fig. 2.1 Stage model of behavioral change according to Lewin

five stagesof behavior change (see Fig. 2.2): 1) Precontemplation stage, 2) Contemplation stage, 3) Preparation stage, 4) Action stage, and 5) Maintenance phase.

1) Precontemplation Phase

The assumption is that individuals generally have no intention of changing their behavior. In this first stage, the current behavior is evaluated and reconsidered. The aim is to initiate a behavior change. A behavior change is only considered when, from the individual's perspective, the current state (e.g., one's weight or high blood pressure) does not match the desired state (e.g., being slim or having normal blood pressure).

2) Contemplation Stagee

In the contemplation stage, considerations for implementing the new behavior are made. The focus is on the formation of an intention. In this stage, people weigh the advantages (e.g., I feel fitter and healthier with less weight) against the disadvantages of the desired behavior (e.g., I have to give up sweets). However, there are no concrete plans for behavior change in this stage yet.

3) Preparation Stage

Concrete plans are developed in the preparation stagee, also known as the planning stage. This stage is about the when and how of performing a behavior. This also includes considerations about difficulties in performing the new behavior (e.g., invitations, business meals, etc.) as well as about one's abilities (e.g., I know which foods are healthy) and the possibility of performing the planned behavior (e.g., is there healthy food in the cafeteria?).

4) Action Stage

In the action stage, the actual implementation of the target behavior plays a central role. Individuals make decisions about when and how which part of the behavior change will be implemented (e.g., I always go to a fitness training on Mondays and Wednesdays).

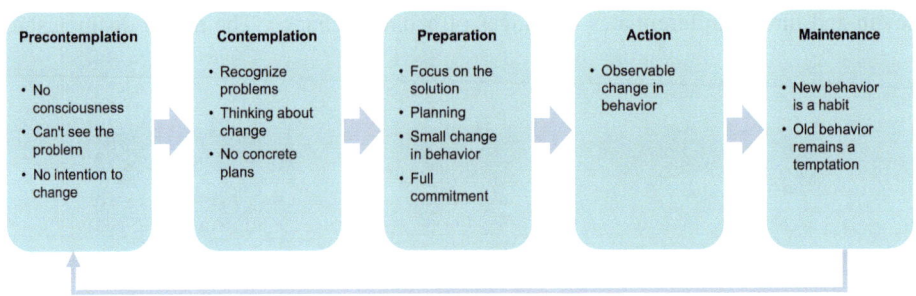

Fig. 2.2 Transtheoretical Model of Behavior Change (Prochaska & Velicer, 1997, p. 39)

5) Maintenance Stage

In the last stage, the maintenance stage, the aim is to establish a new habit. The old behavior is still a temptation and there are relapses into old behavior patterns (e.g., binge eating or skipping exercise units). In this stage, individuals face the challenge of overcoming obstacles, processing failures, and resisting temptations.

A central assumption of the stagemodels of behavior change is that measures for behavior change must be adapted to the stage in which the individual currently is. This means that different measures are relevant for those affected who are not yet aware of the problem than for those who are aware of the problem but fail to actually implement their behavior. For example, individuals in the precontemplation stage need to be informed about the danger of being overweight; individuals in the preparation stage, on the other hand, need support in planning the behavior (e.g., how can I specifically change my diet).

This logic of the connection between the process of behavior change and suitable measures is also applied to the project at hand.

2.1.2 COM-B Model of Behavior Change

In psychology, there are various causal models of behavior. An example of a causal model is the Theory of Planned Behavior by Ajzen (1991). These models explain the causes of behavior and thus serve to explain behavior change. The COM-B model is a causal model and focuses on behavior changes in the health sector (Michie et al., 2011a).

In the COM-B model, **C**apability, **O**pportunity, and **M**otivation interact to explain a **B**ehavior (see Fig. 2.3; Michie et al., 2011). *Capability* is defined as the psychological and physical ability and competence of the individual to perform the relevant activity. Psychological capabilities are the required cognitive processes, memory processes as well as knowledge (e.g., knowledge about which foods are healthy). Physical skills include the ability to perform a desired behavior (e.g., someone can cook healthily). *Motivation* is defined as all neural processes that stimulate and control behavior. These processes can be further divided into reflective and automatic processes: Reflective processes include goals and conscious decisions, automatic processes are habits and emotional reactions. *Opportunity* refers to all factors that lie outside the individual and enable or trigger behavior. These are contextual factors such as the availability of healthy food or time resources to engage in physical activity. The arrows in Fig. 2.3 represent possible influences between the components of the model. For example, opportunity can influence motivation as well as capability. Conversely, the performance of a behavior can also change capability, motivation, and opportunity.

This causal model of behavior provides a basis for selecting and designing activities aimed at behavior change. It offers the possibility to define, for a specific behavior in a specific context, to what extent the adjustment of certain components or combinations

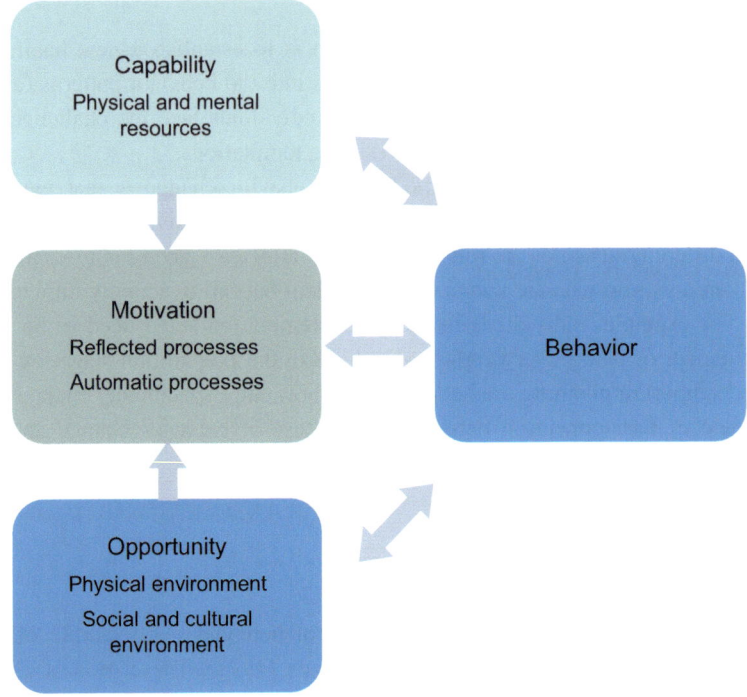

Fig. 2.3 COM-B Model of Behavior Change in the Health Sector (Michie & van Stralen et al., 2011b, p. 4)

of components can lead to the required behavior change. When selecting and designing activities based on the model, it should be taken into account that the causal connections within the model can reduce or enhance the effect of certain measures by leading to changes elsewhere.

2.2   Definition and Classification of Behavior Change Techniques

Understanding the process of behavior change forms the starting point for considerations on how the process can be influenced with regard to a change to a healthy lifestyle. First, clarity should be created about the terminology and, building on this, a classification of behavior change techniques should be made.

2.2.1   Definition of Key Terms

For the present work, the definition of the terms *Intervention, Behavior Change Technique,* and *Measure* is necessary. Fig. 2.4 graphically represents the definition of these three terms.

Intervention: Interventions are a coordinated set of activities aimed at changing specific behavior patterns (Michie & van Stralen et al., 2011b). It is a collective term for a combination of interacting activities. Examples are activities for switching to a healthy diet or activities for integrating more exercise into everyday life. Therefore, interventions are complex and their effect can only be systematically investigated based on the effect of the individual components.

Behavior Change Technique (BCT): A behavior change technique is an observable, replicable, and irreducible component of an intervention. Behavior change techniques aim to influence causal processes that regulate behavior (Michie et al., 2013). Irreducible means that behavior change techniques can be implemented on their own. However, they can also be used in combination. An example of a behavior change technique is setting goals for healthy meals.

Measure: A measure is the concrete design and implementation of the behavior change technique. For example, the specific goal can be to eat only three healthy meals per day. This is the implementation of the behavior change technique of goal setting.

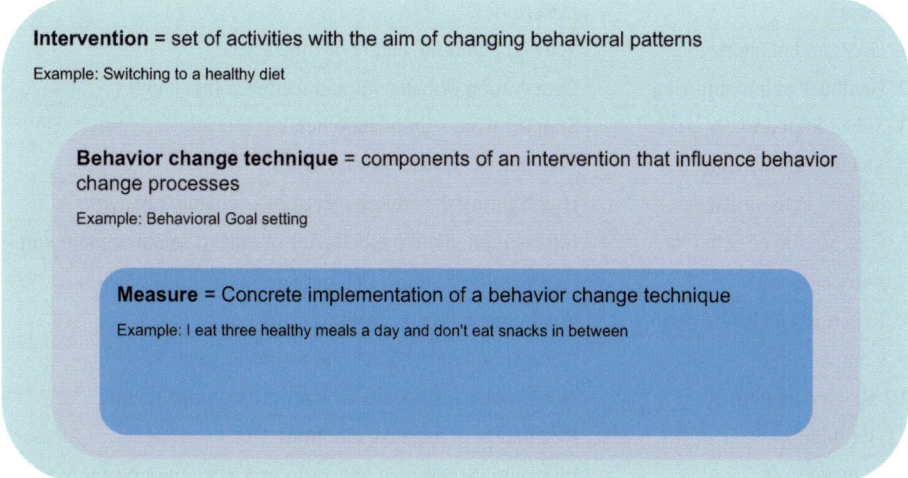

Fig. 2.4 Definition of Key Terms

2.2.2   Classification of Behavior Change Techniques

In light of the growing number of behavior change techniques, one direction of health psychology research is concerned with the classification of these techniques. The most prominent classification is based on the taxonomy by Michie et al. (2013). This served as the starting point for a detailed explanation of behavior change techniques in the present project.

The taxonomy was developed based on a Delphi study with experts in health psychology. The experts were tasked with evaluating 93 behavior change techniques collected from efficacy studies in relation to various dimensions. Based on the evaluations of the experts, the 93 behavior change techniques were clustered into 16 categories (or *clusters* according to Michie et al., 2013) (see Table 2.1).

The numbering in the table and in the explanations corresponds to the official numbering according to the taxonomy by Michie et al. (2013). The 16 categories each include several behavior change techniques, which are explained in the following tables.

Behavior change techniques concerning*Goals and planning (1)* include nine different techniques related to setting, implementing, and reviewing goals (see Table 2.2). In particular, the distinction between goals at the level of behavior (e.g., physical activity) and at the level of outcomes (e.g., weight loss) is important.

Table 2.1   16 categories of behavior change techniques with examples

Category	Description
1. Goals and planning	Setting, planning, and reviewing goals
2. Feedback and monitoring	Observation of behavior and feedback on changes
3. Social Support	Support from significant others
4. Shaping knowledge	Transfer of knowledge and skills
5. Natural consequences	Highlighting the consequences of unhealthy behavior
6. Comparison of behavior	Information about the behavior of others; social comparison
7. Associations	Establishing a connection between a cue and behavior
8. Repetition and substitution	Practicing behavior, building habits
9. Comparison of outcomes	Comparison of behavior and its consequences
10. Reward and threat	Notification and receipt of a reward or punishment
11. Regulation	Regulation of negative emotions
12. Antedecents	Improving situational factors to make behavior easier to show
13. Identity	Activating or improving self-perception
14. Scheduled consequences	Planning rewards and punishments
15. Self-belief	Improving self-confidence in one's own abilities
16. Covert learning	Mental visualization of the consequences of behavior

Table 2.2 Behavior change techniques in Category 1: Goals and planning

No.	Behavior change technique	Description	Example
1.1	Goal setting (behavior)	Goal that describes a behavior	*Run five kilometers every day*
1.2	Problem solving	Analyze behavior and develop strategies to overcome obstacles in pursuing goals	*Since one is too tired to exercise after work in the evening, one plans to exercise in the morning*
1.3	Goal setting (outcome)	Goal that describes an outcome	*Lose two kilos within a month*
1.4	Action planning	Detailed planning of the behavior	*Go running every Monday morning from 8:00–8:45*
1.5	Review behavior goal(s)	Review behavioral goal and adjust if necessary (adjust same goal or set new goal)	*Because the original goal was too ambitious, it is adjusted to running three times a week*
1.6	Discrepancy between current behavior and goal	Record differences between current behavior and behavioral goal, outcome goal, or action planning	*Currently, one goes running twice a week. However, the goal was to go running three times a week*
1.7	Review outcome goal(s)	Review outcome goal and adjust if necessary (adjust same goal or set new goal)	*Within a month, one has lost three kilos. Due to the success, the goal for the next month is adjusted and aimed to lose four kilos*
1.8	Behavioral contract	Record behavioral goal in writing together with a professional	*Record the running goals together with a fitness trainer*
1.9	Commitment	Verbal confirmation of behavioral goals	*Tell oneself that one will definitely go running three times a week*

In the category *Feedback and monitoring (2)*, seven different behavior change techniques are summarized (see Table 2.3). These include various forms of observation and recording of changes as well as corresponding feedback. Here too, the distinction between change at the level of behavior (e.g., physical activity) and at the level of outcomes (e.g., weight loss) is important.

Strategies of *Social support (3)* are behavior change techniques that involve the support of other persons in some form (see Table 2.4). These include different groups of people such as friends, family, work colleagues, or peers.

The category *Shaping knowledge (4)* includes strategies for providing comprehensive knowledge and skills to implement a behavior change (see Table 2.5). This also involves a profound understanding of one's own behavior and the underlying factors of behavior.

Table 2.3 Behavior change techniques in category 2: Feedback and monitoring

No.	Behavior change technique	Description	Example
2.1	Monitoring of behavior by others without feedback	Behavior is recorded by an external person, e.g., health professional (without feedback)	*The nutritionist uses a questionnaire to assess how healthy the eating habits are*
2.2	Feedback on behavior	Purely informative feedback on behaviors	*Feedback on healthy eating habits based on a question-naire*
2.3	Self-monitoring of behavior	Behavior is recorded by the person themselves	*Diary with the meals consumed daily*
2.4	Self-monitoring of outcome(s) of behavior	Results of behavior changes are recorded by the person themselves	*Diary with monthly measurement of body weight*
2.5	Monitoring of of outcome(s) of behavior by others without feedback	Results of behavior changes are recorded by an external person, e.g., health professional (without feedback)	*Doctor measures body weight at each visit*
2.6	Biofeedback	Feedback on physiological parameters	*Doctor measures blood pressure and provides feedback*
2.7	Feedback on outcome(s) of behavior	Feedback on the results of behavior changes	*Doctor provides feedback on the amount of weight loss*

Table 2.4 Behavior change techniques in Category 3: Social support

No.	Behavior change technique	Description	Example
3.1	Social support (unspecified)	Arrange social support or provide information about it	*Appoint a friend as a "buddy" who supports in losing weight*
3.2	Social support (practical)	Practical support for behavior change from other person	*Go jogging twice a week with friends*
3.3	Social support (emotional)	Emotional support for behavior change from other person	*Partner buys flowers and says "You're doing great!"*

The category *Natural consequences (5)* combines behavior change techniques that highlight the consequences of unhealthy behaviors (see Table 2.6). This includes health, social, and emotional impacts.

Table 2.5 Behavior change techniques in category 4: Shaping knowledge

No.	Behavior change technique	Description	Example
4.1	Instruction on how to perform a behavior	Providing specific skills to perform a behavior	*Fitness instructor shows simple fitness exercises for home*
4.2	Information about antecedents	Providing information about factors that influence the relevant behavior	*Information that negative feelings can lead to unhealthy eating behavior*
4.3	Re-attribution	Determining the perceived causes of behavior and suggesting alternative explanations	*Recognizing that a person does not eat too much because they like to eat, but because they have forgotten how to properly perceive hunger*
4.4	Behavioral experiments	Investigating the influence of causes and behaviors with data	*Monitoring cholesterol levels after a stage with predominantly animal protein and after a stage with predominantly plant protein*

Table 2.6 Behavior change techniques in Category 5: Natural consequences

No.	Behavior change technique	Description	Example
5.1	Information about health consequences	Provide information about the health consequences of behaviors	*Obesity can lead to Type II diabetes*
5.2	Salience of consequences	Emphasize the consequences of unhealthy behaviors so they are better remembered	*Type II diabetes often leads to severe foot wounds*
5.3	Information about social and environmental consequences	Provide information about the social and environmental consequences of behaviors	*When a person is fitter again, they can go on hiking trips with friends*
5.4	Monitoring of emotional consequences	Assessment of the feelings one has after showing the behavior	*Keep a diary about how you feel after you have been jogging*
5.5	Anticipated regret	Raise awareness of future regret for undesired behaviors	*Imagine how you would feel if you haven't gone running for two weeks*
5.6	Information about emotional consequences	Provide information about the emotional consequences of behaviors	*After a run, you are relaxed and feel physically well*

The category *Comparison of behavior (6)* is about information on other people's behavior and social comparisons (see Table 2.7).

The behavior change techniques from the category *Associations (7)* aim to establish connections between cues and desired behaviors or to reduce the connection to undesired behaviors (see Table 2.8).

The category *Repetition and substitution (8)* is about practicing new, healthy behaviors (see Table 2.9). The focus thereby is on the development of habits.

The category *Comparison of outcomes (9)* includes behavior change techniques where arguments for and against a behavior and the corresponding effects are compared (see Table 2.10).

The category *Reward and threat (10)* involves rewards for desired behavior and punishments (in a broader sense) for undesired behavior (see Table 2.11). It distinguishes between the announcement of a future reward and the actual receipt of a reward. Furthermore, it differentiates between different forms of rewards: material, social, or nonspecific rewards.

The category *Regulation (11)* concerns emotion regulation in the face of negative emotions and stress (see Table 2.12).

The category *Antedecents (12)*t is about changing situational factors so that the desired behavior can be carried out more easily, or the undesired behavior is made more difficult (see Table 2.13).

The category *Identity (13)* describes behavior change techniques in which self-perception is activated or altered (see Table 2.14). This category also includes techniques in which the perception of the desired behavior is altered.

The category *Scheduled consequences (14)* involves agreeing on rewards for desired behavior and punishments (in a broader sense) for undesired behavior (see Table 2.15). The types of reward and punishment referred to in category 14 are described in category 10 Reward and threat.

Table 2.7 Behavior change techniques in Category 6: Comparison of behavior

No.	Behavior change technique	Description	Example
6.1	Demonstration of the behavior	Provide an example of someone showing the desired behavior, e.g. in person or via film (learning by modelling)	*Reading a blog of a person affected to get inspiration on how to incorporate exercise into everyday life*
6.2	Social comparison	Encourage comparison with other people	*Compare weight loss with other affected people*
6.3	Information about others' approval	Information about what other people think about the behavior	*In the village, it is appreciated when one is actively involved in the gymnastics club*

Table 2.8 Behavior change techniques in category 7: Associations

No.	Behavior change technique	Description	Example
7.1	Prompts/ Cues	Establish a social or environmental stimulus that triggers the desired behavior	*Place a yoga mat in front of the bed so that you start the morning with a yoga session*
7.2	Cues signallingreward	Establish an environmental stimulus that announces a reward	*After 30 minutes of fitness training, calm music comes on, announcing the final relaxation*
7.3	Reduce prompts/cues	Gradually reduce the stimulus that triggers the desired behavior	*Gradually place the yoga mat in front of the bed less often*
7.4	Remove access to the reward	Avoid situations where undesired behavior is rewarded	*Not having sweets in the house*
7.5	Remove aversive stimulus	Arrange a negative stimulus that is removed when the desired behavior is performed	*A buddy who constantly asks if you are finally going to the gym together*
7.6	Satiation	Connection to the undesired behavior is reduced by repeated exposure to a cue	*Always go through the candy aisle when shopping until the habit of buying something stops*
7.7	Exposure	Confrontation with a feared stimulus to reduce a later negative reaction	*Show and explain the tools at a health check-up (e.g., syringe for blood draw) to reduce fear of doctor visits*
7.8	Associative learning	Combine a neutral stimulus with a stimulus that triggers the desired behavior until the desired behavior is triggered by the neutral stimulus (classical conditioning)	*Drink coffee on the yoga mat in the morning until coffee is automatically associated with yoga*

The category *Self-belief (15)* describes behavior change techniques aimed at strengthening self-confidence in one's own abilities and self-efficacy (see Table 2.16).

The category *Covert learning (16)* is about learning by imagining the positive and negative consequences of behavior (see Table 2.17).

The effectiveness of various behavior change techniques in relation to the adoption of a healthy lifestyle is presented in the following section based on meta-analyses.

Table 2.9 Behavior change techniques in category 8: Repetition and substitution

No.	Behavior change technique	Description	Example
8.1	Behavioral practice/rehearsal	Practice behaviors in a safe environment	*Practice simple fitness exercises with a fitness instructor*
8.2	Behavior substitution	Replace unwanted behavior with desired or neutral behavior	*Eat an orange instead of a pastry with coffee*
8.3	Habit formation	Repeatedly perform behavior in the same context until it becomes a habit	*Do ten minutes of yoga every morning after coffee*
8.4	Habit reversal	Replace unwanted habit with a new, healthier habit	*Always take the stairs instead of the elevator on the way to the office*
8.5	Overcorrection	Perform desired behavior excessively after unwanted behavior has been shown	*If too many sweets have been eaten, then eat no sweets at all for a while*
8.6	Generalization of a target behavior	Perform desired behavior, which is already shown in certain situations, in other situations as well	*Not only take the stairs on the way to the office, but everywhere*
8.7	Graded tasks	Start with simple tasks and make them increasingly difficult until the desired behavior is shown	*Start with fast walks, then small jogging rounds, until the person can do five kilometers*

Table 2.10 Behavior change techniques in Category 9: Comparison of outcomes

No.	Behavior change technique	Description	Example
9.1	Credible source	Information (for or against the behavior) from a credible source	*Video from a well-known and popular health expert emphasizing the importance of daily exercise*
9.2	Pros and cons	Collect and compare arguments for and against a behavior change	*Pro and con list for regular jogging rounds*
9.3	Comparative imagining of future outcomes	Imagine and compare the future with and without behavior change	*Imagine where you will be in two years if you seek nutritional counseling or if you do not*

Table 2.11 Behavior change techniques in Category 10: Reward and threat

No.	Behavior change technique	Description	Example
10.1	Material incentive (behavior)	Information about receiving a financial or material reward for the desired behavior	*If you go jogging three times a week, you will receive a voucher for sportswear*
10.2	Material reward (behavior)	Receiving a financial or material reward for the desired behavior	*Receiving a voucher for sportswear after jogging three times a week*
10.3	Non-specific reward	Receiving an unspecified reward for the desired behavior	*Receiving a nice outing after jogging three times a week*
10.4	Social reward	Receiving a verbal or non-verbal social reward for the desired behavior	*Receiving a "Well-done" sticker after jogging three times a week*
10.5	Social incentive	Information about receiving a verbal or non-verbal social reward for the desired behavior	*If you go jogging three times a week, will you receive a "Well-done" sticker*
10.6	Non-specific incentive	Information about receiving an unspecified reward for the desired behavior	*If you go jogging three times a week, you will receive a nice outing*
10.7	Self-incentive	Planning to reward oneself for the desired behavior	*If you go jogging, you treat yourself to a bubble bath afterwards*
10.8	Incentive (outcome)	Information about receiving a reward for the desired outcome	*If you lose five kilos, you will receive a wellness voucher*
10.9	Self-reward	Rewarding oneself for the desired behavior	*Treating oneself to a bubble bath after jogging*
10.10	Reward (outcome)	Receiving a reward for the desired outcome	*Receiving a wellness voucher after losing five kilos*
10.11	Future punishment	Information about future punishment or omission of rewards if the undesired behavior is shown	*If you do not regularly go to the gym, the support for the gym subscription is dropped*

Table 2.12 Behavior change techniques in category 11: Regulation

No.	Behavior change technique	Description	Example
11.1	Pharmacological support	Promote or maintain medication intake	*Visit a general practitioner to receive medicinal support for high blood pressure*
11.2	Reduce negative emotions	Recommendation of ways to reduce negative emotions that hinder showing the behavior	*Join a group like Weight Watchers to discuss how to deal with setbacks*
11.3	Conserving mental resources	Recommendation of ways to reduce mental effort that hinders showing the behavior	*Recommendation of healthy recipes that make it easier to prepare a healthy meal*
11.4	Paradoxical interventions	Recommendation to intensify the *undesirable* behavior with the aim of it losing its appeal	*The person should eat ten sweets every day*

Table 2.13 Behavior change techniques in category 12: Antedecents

No.	Behavior change technique	Description	Example
12.1	Restructuring the physical environment	Design the physical environment in a way that the desired behavior can be carried out more easily	*Place the bicycle directly in front of the house (instead of in the basement) to make it easier to go shopping by bike*
12.2	Restructuring the social environment	Design the social environment in a way that the desired behavior can be carried out more easily	*Maintain friendships with people who place a lot of value on physical activity and exercise*
12.3	Avoidance/reducing exposure to cues for the behavior	Avoid or reduce exposure to physical and social stimuli that trigger undesired behavior	*Reduce restaurant visits with friends if they encourage unhealthy eating and excessive drinking*
12.4	Distraction	Focus attention on something other than the trigger for undesired behavior	*In the cafeteria, focus on the colorful salad bar instead of looking at the cake counter*
12.5	Adding objects to the environment	Place objects in the environment that facilitate the desired behavior	*Set up a trampoline in the living room to take regular active breaks*
12.6	Body changes	Improve physical abilities from within (e.g., physiotherapy) or with external support (e.g., medical aid)	*Do strength training to strengthen muscles for more physical activity*

Table 2.14 Behavior change techniques in category 13: Identity

No.	Behavior change technique	Description	Example
13.1	Identification of self as role model	Self-perception as a role model for others	*Eating healthily because you want to be a good role model for your children*
13.2	Framing/reframing	Change perception of behavior to change associated thoughts and feelings	*Short walks during work are good for new ideas (and not just for more exercise)*
13.3	Incompatible beliefs	Focus on discrepancies between behavior and self-perception (cognitive dissonance)	*Perception that you never exercise, although you are actually an active person*
13.4	Valued self-identity	Emphasize a personally important value or personal strength (e.g., by writing it down)	*Write down that you are a person who likes to move in nature and in the fresh air*
13.5	Identity associated with changed behavior	Construction of a self-perception that is defined by the changed behavior	*Perceive yourself as a person who used to be a junk food fan, but now values a healthy diet*

2.3 Effectiveness of Behavior Change Techniques in the Prevention of Overweight and Diabetes

The analysis of the effectiveness of behavior change techniques is a central research area of health psychology. Numerous individual studies and meta-analyses deal with the effectiveness of behavior change techniques in the prevention and treatment of overweight, hypertension, and diabetes (Cradock, ÓLaighin, Finucane, Cradock, ÓLaighin et al., 2017; Gainforth, et al., 2017; Hankonen et al., 2015; Lara et al., 2014; McEwan et al., 2019; Samdal et al., 2017). These generally clinical randomized control trials measure the effect of behavior change techniques on objectively measurable factors (e.g., relative weight reduction, blood sugar reduction).

Behavior change techniques are active components of the interventions in these medically oriented studies, i.e., they change, regulate, and direct behavior, which serves the implementation of a healthy lifestyle. The central medical interventions are changes in diet (e.g., reduction of the number of calories, skipping meals, proteins instead of carbohydrates, etc.) and an increase in exercise (e.g., sports programs, exercise units). The effectiveness of these medical interventions has been demonstrated multiple times in large-scale studies (see overview study by Cradock, ÓLaighin, Finucane, Gainforth et al., 2017). However, it has also been shown that the initial effect of these medical interventions quickly diminishes (Kwasnicka et al., 2016). The central question of

Table 2.15 Behavior change techniques in category 14: Scheduled consequences

No.	Behavior change technique	Description	Example
14.1	Behavior cost	Removal of a reward for undesirable behavior	*If you don't go to yoga three times a week, you have to repay the gym voucher*
14.2	Punishment	Punishment in a broader sense for undesirable behavior	*If you don't go to yoga three times a week, you have to do all the housework*
14.3	Remove reward	Removal of an existing reward for undesirable behavior	*If you don't go to yoga three times a week, you are not allowed to go to the sauna as a reward, as usual*
14.4	Reward approximation	Reward for approaching the goal, with the bar gradually being raised	*First, you go to the sauna after every yoga session, then after every second one, then after every third one, etc.*
14.5	Rewarding completion	Reward for achieving the goal and gradually including previous steps in the reward	*Reward for healthy takeaway food, then for healthy, home-cooked food, then for healthy, home-cooked food with exclusively fresh ingredients*
14.6	Situation-specific reward	Reward in one situation, but not in another situation	*Reward for eating during defined meal times and not in between*
14.7	Reward incompatible behavior	Reward for new behavior that differs from previous behavior in this situation	*Reward for ordering a Poké Bowl in the restaurant, instead of always ordering fries with schnitzel as before*
14.8	Reward alternative behavior	Reward for alternative behavior to the undesirable behavior	*Reward for going to the cinema instead of the pub*
14.9	Reduce reward frequency	Link reward with increased frequency or duration	*Reward if you go to yoga once a week, then if you go twice a week, etc.*
14.10	Remove punishment	Removal of unpleasant consequence when desired behavior is shown	*If you go to yoga three times a week, the partner takes over all the housework*

Table 2.16   Behavior change techniques in category 15: Self-belief

No.	Behavior change technique	Description	Example
15.1	Verbal persuasion about capability	Encouraging and convincing the patient that they can implement the desired behavior	*Reassuring the patient that she is an open and committed person who will be able to implement new eating habits*
15.2	Mental rehearsal of successful performance	Imagining and practicing new behaviors mentally	*Imagining how to put together a rich salad from the counter during lunch break*
15.3	Focus on past success	Thinking about and/or listing past successes	*Thinking about past lunches in the cafeteria where you always chose a salad*
15.4	Self-talk	Positive self-talk or thoughts before/during the desired behavior	*Looking forward to the lunch where you can put together a delicious salad*

Table 2.17   Behavior change techniques in category 16: Covert learning

No.	Behavior change technique	Description	Example
16.1	Imaginary punishment	Imagining the unwanted behavior and the subsequent punishment	*Imagining how you feel after eating a huge portion of fries and schnitzel*
16.2	Imaginary reward	Imagining the desired behavior and the subsequent reward	*Imagining how you feel after attending a yoga class*
16.3	Vicarious consequences	Observing the consequences of behavior and the subsequent reward/punishment in others	*Observing how relaxed the participants return from the yoga class*

effectiveness research is which of the behavior change techniques support a *sustainable* behavior change.

The meta-analysis by Cradlock et al. (2017) shows which behavior change techniques are frequently used. According to this overview study, the most widespread behavior change techniques are the following: 1) Instruction on how to perform a behavior, 2) credible source, 3) self-monitoring of behavior, 4) monitoring of behavior by others without feedback, 5) goal setting (behavior), 6) social support (unspecified), 7) adding objects to the environment.

Following, the results of the effect of behavior change techniques from various meta-analyses are presented. Studies focusing on weight reduction show that behavior change techniques from all 16 categories have a significant influence on weight reduction (Hankonen et al., 2015; McEwan et al., 2019). The meta-analysis by Hankonen et al. (2015) demonstrates that it is the actual application of the behavior change techniques by the affected individuals that leads to a demonstrable effect of the interventions. The study by McEwan et al. (2019) shows that the effect of behavior change techniques is stronger when they are implemented in the understanding of the literature-based definition.

Meta-analyses with effectiveness measures based on medical factors (blood sugar levels HbA_{1c}) present a more differentiated picture. Table 2.18 shows which behavior change techniques have led to significant medical effects in meta-analyses. These effects refer to a period of three to six months.

The meta-analysis in the field of nutrition presents a slightly different picture. Here, the behavior change techniques listed in Table 2.19 are effective in relation to the consumption of fruits and vegetables. Since a different taxonomy for classifying behavior change techniques was used in the meta-analysis by Lara et al. (2014), the CALO-RE taxonomy (Michie et al., 2011a, b, c), these were assigned based on their description to the taxonomy used in Sect. 2.2.2 (Michie et al., 2013). Particularly effective are the behavior change techniques of problem solving and social support. The study further shows that the more behavior change techniques are applied, the greater the effect. This underlines the relevance of combining different behavior change techniques. A meta-analysis in the field of overweight comes to similar results (Samdal et al., 2017).

Table 2.18 Significant effects of behavior change techniques on blood sugar reduction

Behavior change technique	Dependent variable	Area of behavior change	Reference
1.2 Problem solving	HbA_{1c}	Nutrition	(Cradock et al., 2017a)
1.4 Action planning	HbA_{1c}	Nutrition, Exercise	(Cradock et al., 2017b)
2.2 Feedback on behavior	HbA_{1c}	Nutrition	(Cradock et al., 2017a)
4.1 Instruction on how to perform the behavior	HbA_{1c}	Nutrition, Exercise	(Cradock et al., 2017b)
6.1 Demonstration of the behavior	HbA_{1c}	Nutrition, Exercise	(Cradock et al., 2017b)
6.2 Social comparison	HbA_{1c}	Nutrition	(Cradock et al., 2017a)
8.1 Behavioral practice/ rehearsal	HbA_{1c}	Nutrition, Exercise	(Cradock et al., 2017b)
12.5 Adding objects to the environment	HbA1c; Nutrition	HbA1c; Nutrition	(Cradock et al., 2017a)

Table 2.19 Significant effects of behavior change techniques on nutrition, overweight, and exercise

Behavior change technique	Area of behavior change	Meta-analysis
1.1 Goal setting (behavior)	Nutrition, overweight, and exercise	(Samdal et al., 2017)
1.2 Problem solving	Nutrition (consumption of fruits and vegetables)	(Lara et al., 2014)
1.3 Goal setting (outcome)	Nutrition (consumption of fruits and vegetables), over-weight, and exercise	(Lara et al., 2014; Samdal et al., 2017)
2.3 Self-monitoring of behavior	Nutrition, overweight, and exercise	(Samdal et al., 2017)
2.7 Feedback on outcome(s) of behavior	Nutrition (consumption of fruits and vegetables), over-weight, and exercise	(Lara et al., 2014; Samdal et al., 2017)
3.1 Social support (unspecified)	Nutrition (consumption of fruits and vegetables)	(Lara et al., 2014)
7.3 Reduce prompts/cues	Nutrition (consumption of fruits and vegetables)	(Lara et al., 2014)
8.7 Graded tasks	Nutrition, overweight, and exercise	(Samdal et al., 2017)
12.5 Adding objects to the environment	Nutrition, overweight, and exercise	(Samdal et al., 2017)

It must be noted as a limitation that the overview of the effect of behavior change techniques based on meta-analyses presents a mixed picture. This is due to various problems in measuring the effectiveness of behavior change techniques. Firstly, the effectiveness depends on the specific design of a measure. For example, goal setting can be implemented in different ways. Secondly, the treatment fidelity can vary greatly, i.e., the individuals can adhere more or less well to the instructions. These factors are difficult to control in meta-analyses and therefore lead to different results in terms of effectiveness.

Another point of criticism of effectiveness analyses is their time horizon. The overview studies with medical effect data cannot prove a sustainable behavior change. The studies on behavior change in the field of nutrition and exercise are either designed for a shorter time horizon (max. twelve months) or make no statement about the time horizon.

Overall, however, the meta-analyses show that all behavior change techniques listed in section 2.2 successfully contribute to the effect of interventions in the field of nutrition and exercise. The proven effect can only be demonstrated for short time horizons. In the long term—as far as this point has been investigated—there is no evidence of an effect for all behavior change techniques. This brings the central question of the present project back into focus: How can motivation be maintained to implement behavior change techniques in the long term and thus maintain a behavior change?

2.4   Motivation and Self-Management

From a theoretical perspective, two groups of approaches to maintaining new behavior can be distinguished (Kwasnicka et al., 2016): The first group (e.g. the theory of planned behavior or the COM-B model) assumes that the same factors are relevant for maintaining a new behavior as for its initiation. The second group of theoretical approaches goes beyond this assumption and is based on a more differentiated basis: These approaches postulate that different factors are relevant for maintenance than for initial implementation. From this second group of theories, five overarching factors influencing the maintenance of behavior changes can be identified based on a meta-analysis (Kwasnicka et al., 2016):

1. Motivation
2. Self-regulation
3. Psychological and physical resources
4. Habits
5. Contextual influences

Motivation and self-regulation emerge as central overarching psychological factors for a sustainable behavior change. On this basis, the present project will place a special focus on these factors. Subsequently, both factors will be briefly explained in the context of maintaining behavior changes in the health sector and will be integrated in the empirical studies. The other factors *psychological and physical resources, habits* and *contextual influences* will only be dealt with marginally in the present project.

2.4.1 Motivation

The Self-Determination Theory (SDT) by Deci and Ryan (2000) serves to explain the influence of motivation on the maintenance of new behavior. SDT focuses not on the quantity, but on the quality of motivation (Hagger et al., 2020). In this context, SDT distinguishes between intrinsic and extrinsic motivation. Intrinsic motivation refers to intentional behavior due to enjoyment of the behavior itself, personal benefits from it, or alignment with personal values. In contrast, in the case of extrinsic motivation behavior occurs due to reward, social pressure, or to avoid feelings of guilt (Sheeran et al., 2016).

Intrinsic and extrinsic motivation differ in perceived causality: Intrinsic motivation is based on autonomous motives, i.e., a behavior is perceived as voluntary and shown out of one's own volition, e.g., for the enjoyment of the behavior itself. In contrast, extrinsic motivation is based on controlled motives, i.e., behavior is perceived as imposed from the outside and performed due to an external force, e.g., due to a reward. Autonomous and controlled motives represent a continuum, and there are different mixed forms that contain both types of motivation in varying degrees (see Fig. 2.5). In *Integrated regulation*, a behavior that was previously carried out due to controlled motives is internalized and subsequently perceived as autonomously motivated. *Identified regulation* means, that a behavior is carried out because it is perceived as valuable or important. In *Introjected regulation*, a behavior is carried out to maintain self-esteem or appreciation by others. *Amotivation* is represented outside the continuum because in this state a behavior is carried out without reason or goal—thus without any motives.

The meta-analysis by Sheeran et al. (2016) shows that an increase in intrinsic motivation is associated with successful behavior change in the health sector. Based on this finding, it is assumed that behavior change techniques that are oriented towards intrinsic motivation support the effectiveness of medical interventions and thus promote the maintenance of behavior changes. This assumption forms an important basis for the empirical study, which is described in detail in Chap. 5.

2.4.2   Self-Management

Approaches to self-management or self-regulation assume that those affected can maintain a behavior change if they successfully monitor the results of the new behavior (monitoring) and have effective strategies to overcome barriers associated with performing the new, desired behavior.

Self-regulation processes are defined as "processes that serve to control or steer thoughts, feelings, and actions to achieve goals. These processes include dynamic iterations of goal setting, planning and implementation of behaviors, evaluation of progress

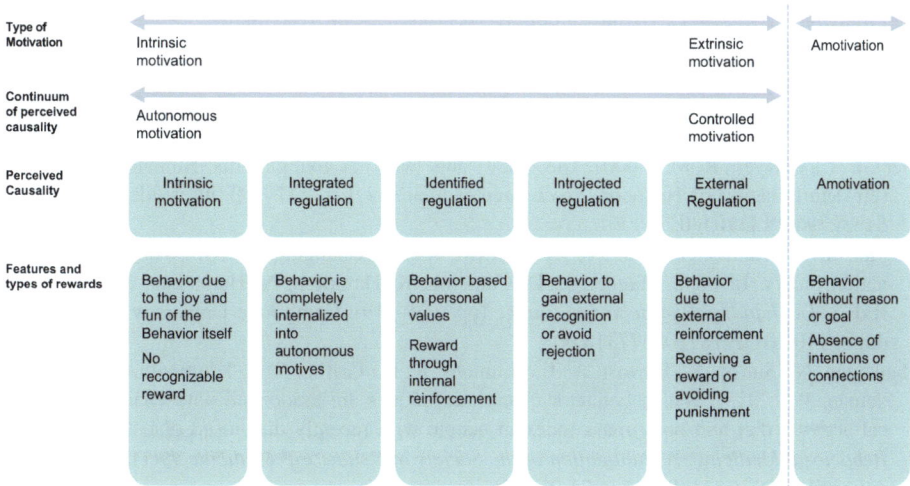

Fig. 2.5 Intrinsic and extrinsic motivation and perceived causality (Hagger et al., 2020, p. 106)

in achieving goals, and corresponding revision of goals and actions." (Cameron et al., 2020, p. 60). Self-regulation is based on the principles of control theory, which defines behavior as constant change to move one's own current state towards one's own goals, norms, and ideals (Cameron et al., 2020, p. 60). In addition, emotional processes are of central relevance in self-regulation. These are processes that explain how emotions affect behavior: Negative emotions as well as positive emotions motivate behavior. An example is the fear of diseases that motivate people to take protective measures such as dietary adjustments (Cameron et al., 2020, p. 60).

Self-management is defined—with reference to the principles of self-regulation—as a higher-level therapeutic principle that is supposed to support people in controlling their own behavior according to their own goal representations. The aim of self-management is self-regulation and autonomy.

References

Ajzen, I. (1991). The theory of planned behavior. *Organizational Behavior and Human Decision Processes,50*(2), 179–211. https://doi.org/10.1016/0749-5978(91)90020-T.

Bamberg, S. (2012). Wie funktioniert Verhaltensänderung?: Das MAX-Selbstregulationsmodell. In U. Reutter & M. Stiewe (Eds.), *Mobilitätsmanagement: Wissenschaftliche Grundlagen und Wirkungen in der Praxis* (pp. 76–101). Klartext.

Cameron, L. D., Fleszar-Pavlović, S., & Khachikian, T. (2020). Changing behavior using the common sense model of self-regulation. In M. S. Hagger, L. D. Cameron, K. Hamilton, N. Hankonen, & T. Lintunen (Eds.), *The handbook of behavior change* (pp. 60–76). Cambridge University Press. https://doi.org/10.1017/9781108677318.005.

Cradock, K. A., ÓLaighin, G., Finucane, F. M., Gainforth, H. L., Quinlan, L. R., & Ginis, K. A. M. (2017a). Behaviour change techniques targeting both diet and physical activity in type 2 diabetes: A systematic review and meta-analysis. *International Journal of Behavioral Nutrition and Physical Activity, 14*(1), 18. https://doi.org/10.1186/s12966-016-0436-0.

Cradock, K. A., ÓLaighin, G., Finucane, F. M., McKay, R., Quinlan, L. R., Martin Ginis, K. A., & Gainforth, H. L. (2017b). Diet behavior change techniques in type 2 diabetes: A systematic review and meta-analysis. *Diabetes Care,40*(12), 1800–1810. https://doi.org/10.2337/dc17-0462.

Deci, E. L., & Ryan, R. M. (2000). The "what" and "why" of goal pursuits: Human needs and the self-determination of behavior. *Psychological Inquiry,11*(4), 227–268. https://doi.org/10.1207/S15327965PLI1104_01.

Hagger, M. S., Hankonen, N. E., & Ryan, R. M. (2020). Changing behavior using self-determination theory. In M. S. Hagger, L. D. Cameron, K. Hamilton, N. Hankonen, & T. Lintunen (Eds.), *The handbook of behavior change* (pp. 104–119). Cambridge University Press. https://doi.org/10.1017/9781108677318.008.

Hankonen, N., Sutton, S., Prevost, A. T., Simmons, R. K., Griffin, S. J., Kinmonth, A. L., & Hardeman, W. (2015). Which behavior change techniques are associated with changes in physical activity, diet and body mass index in people with recently diagnosed diabetes? *Annals of Behavioral Medicine: A Publication of the Society of Behavioral Medicine,49*(1), 7–17. https://doi.org/10.1007/s12160-014-9624-9.

Kwasnicka, D., Dombrowski, S. U., White, M., & Sniehotta, F. (2016). Theoretical explanations for maintenance of behaviour change: A systematic review of behaviour theories. *Health Psychology Review,10*(3), 277–296. https://doi.org/10.1080/17437199.2016.1151372.

Lara, J., Evans, E. H., O'Brien, N., Moynihan, P. J., Meyer, T. D., Adamson, A. J., Errington, L., Sniehotta, F. F., White, M., & Mathers, J. C. (2014). Association of behaviour change techniques with effectiveness of dietary interventions among adults of retirement age: A systematic review and meta-analysis of randomised controlled trials. *BMC Medicine,12*(1), 177. https://doi.org/10.1186/s12916-014-0177-3.

Lewin, K. (1951). *Field theory in social science*. Harper and Row.

McEwan, D., Beauchamp, M. R., Kouvousis, C., Ray, C. M., Wyrough, A., & Rhodes, R. E. (2019). Examining the active ingredients of physical activity interventions underpinned by theory versus no stated theory: A meta-analysis. *Health Psychology Review,13*(1), 1–17. https://doi.org/10.1080/17437199.2018.1547120.

Michie, S., Ashford, S., Sniehotta, F. F., Dombrowski, S. U., Bishop, A., & French, D. P. (2011a). A refined taxonomy of behaviour change techniques to help people change their physical activity and healthy eating behaviours: The CALO-RE taxonomy. *Psychology & Health,26*(11), 1479–1498. https://doi.org/10.1080/08870446.2010.540664.

Michie, S., Hyder, N., Walia, A., & West, R. (2011b). Development of a taxonomy of behaviour change techniques used in individual behavioural support for smoking cessation | Elsevier Enhanced Reader. *Addictive Behaviors,36*(4), 315–319. https://doi.org/10.1016/j.addbeh.2010.11.016.

Michie, S., Richardson, M., Johnston, M., Abraham, C., Francis, J., Hardeman, W., Eccles, M. P., Cane, J., & Wood, C. E. (2013). The behavior change technique taxonomy (v1) of 93 hierarchically clustered techniques: Building an international consensus for the reporting of behavior change interventions. *Annals of Behavioral Medicine,46*(1), 81–95. https://doi.org/10.1007/s12160-013-9486-6.

Michie, S., van Stralen, M. M., & West, R. (2011c). The behaviour change wheel: A new method for characterising and designing behaviour change interventions. *Implementation Science,6*(1), 42. https://doi.org/10.1186/1748-5908-6-42.

Prochaska, J. O., & Velicer, W. F. (1997). The transtheoretical model of health behavior change. *American Journal of Health Promotion,12*(1), 38–48. https://doi.org/10.4278/0890-1171-12.1.38.

Samdal, G. B., Eide, G. E., Barth, T., Williams, G., & Meland, E. (2017). Effective behaviour change techniques for physical activity and healthy eating in overweight and obese adults; systematic review and meta-regression analyses. *International Journal of Behavioral Nutrition and Physical Activity,14*(1), 42. https://doi.org/10.1186/s12966-017-0494-y.

Sheeran, P., Maki, A., Montanaro, E., Avishai-Yitshak, A., Bryan, A., Klein, W. M. P., Miles, E., & Rothman, A. J. (2016). The impact of changing attitudes, norms, and self-efficacy on health-related intentions and behavior: A meta-analysis. *Health Psychology: Official Journal of the Division of Health Psychology, American Psychological Association,35*(11), 1178–1188. https://doi.org/10.1037/hea0000387.

Tversky, A., & Kahneman, D. (1974). Judgment under uncertainty: Heuristics and biases *Science,185*(4157), 1124–1131. https://doi.org/10.1126/science.185.4157.1124.

Basics and Insights from Service Management and Health Economics

3

Contents

Abstract

The scientific discipline of Transformative Service Research (TSR) investigates how the well-being of consumers and society can be improved through services. It aims to contribute to designing and providing services in a way that supports health and society. The field of TSR plays an important role within service research and is used alongside the psychological perspective as a discipline for the present research project. At the same time, questions of quality and efficiency of medical care of non-communicable diseases arise, which are examined from the perspective of health economics. This chapter presents the current state of research from the perspective of these scientific disciplines.

© The Author(s), under exclusive license to Springer-Verlag GmbH, DE, part of Springer   39
Nature 2024
A. Schäfer et al., *Maintaining a Healthy Lifestyle*,
https://doi.org/10.1007/978-3-662-69460-2_3

The well-being of society is addressed in various scientific disciplines. The following Sect. 3.1 provides an overview of the current state of research from the perspective of Transformative Service Research, TSR. Society is made up of individuals. A crucial factor is to consider the change in lifestyle from the perspective of individuals. The viewpoint of the affected persons is therefore analysed with the help of a customer journey (Sect. 3.2). The question of how affected persons can be supported by their environment is examined in greater depth with the help of an ecosystem approach (Sect. 3.3). Finally, the role of the actors in a healthcare system will be presented from a health economics perspective (Sect. 3.4). The focus is on interprofessional cooperation, as this can be expected to lead to improved health outcomes, which in turn benefits the well-being of society.

3.1   Classification of the project in the Transformative Service Research (TSR)

The objective of the Transformative Service Research (TSR) "centers oncreating of uplifting, motivating changes and improvements in the well-being of consumer entities: individuals (consumers and employees), communities and the ecosystem" (Anderson et al., 2011, p. 3). While weight loss can boost well-being at least in the short term, this does not necessarily mean a sustainable lifestyle change, as people who lose weight often quickly regain it (Montani et al., 2015). The sole focus on short-term weight loss is not sufficient from the perspective of the TSR (Taiminen et al., 2020). Rather, the transformative value potential of services that increase wellbeing lies in their ability to bring about lasting change, in the case of the present project, to support the sticking to a healthy lifestyle. The realization of this potential manifests not only in improved well-being, but also in the intention of consumers to maintain the improved well-being (Taiminen et al., 2020).

TSR builds on the theoretical foundations of co-creation and service-dominant logic (SDL) (Kuppelwieser & Finsterwalder, 2016; Previte & Robertson, 2019). It argues that (health) services are an interactive process with the goal of increasing well-being. Co-creation describes the method, process, or result of a collaborative value creation process involving multiple individuals. In marketing and product development, co-creation is a management approach that allows companies and customers to collaborate. This intensive collaboration is intended to achieve better performance and synergy effects. In health services, patients are heavily involved in activities related to the protection and promotion of their well-being. In the context of this research, cocreation can be said to occur, for example, when patients follow the recommendations of service providers (e.g., doctors or pharmacies) and take medication according to the prescribed dosage. This achieves value creation in the form of increased well-being in the sense of co-creation. The SDL assumes that services are provided in value creation processes in which various actors interact as participants. They bring skills and knowledge (operative resources) as well as goods and materials (operand resources) for their own benefit or for the benefit of others into the service network (Vargo & Lusch, 2004, 2008). Co-creation is a key aspect of the SDL.

In an integrated view of SDL and TSR, consumers increase their well-being through the use of services and service providers try to promote the well-being of consumers through appropriate value propositions (Kuppelwieser & Finsterwalder, 2016). Value propositions describe the performance promise to customers and are the reason why they turn to one company rather than another (Osterwalder et al., 2015). Therefore, value propositions (e.g., feeling healthier and being more efficient by adhering to physical activities) can be an important reason that explains why customers use certain services (Chandler & Lusch, 2015).

To support the value proposition of a healthy lifestyle, doctors, nutritionists, and possibly other service providers from the health ecosystem (e.g., pharmacies, health insurance companies) offer measures for those affected. The measures provided serve as a resource for joint value creation. However, they are only successful if the measures (e.g., regular monitoring of physical activities) are utilised and adhered to. This process requires those affected to take responsibility and actively contribute to the service process (Chan et al., 2010; Dellande et al., 2004). They must take control and regularly adjust their behavior to maintain a healthy lifestyle. Under what conditions this succeeds and what the current state of research from the perspective of health psychology is, was explained in Chap. 2 of this book. From the perspective of service research, it is interesting to see which steps and activities those affected go through in the maintenance phase and with or at which contact points of the health ecosystem, so-called touchpoints, they interact (the ecosystem itself is discussed in Sect. 3.3). This touchpoint approach can be analysed using the customer journey explained in Sect. 3.2.

Various studies point to the great importance of social support in the tranistion to a healthy lifestyle (e.g., Ballantine & Stephenson, 2011; Hwang et al., 2010; Parkinson et al., 2017). Social support can come from different people and organizations and, based on House (1981), can have four different dimensions: *informational, instrumental, emotional* and *encouraging* support. The *informational* dimension refers to information, guidelines or advice given by others (e.g., discussions about the calorie content of food as part of nutritional counseling). *Instrumental* support refers to tangible help in the form of resources such as money, materials or work (e.g., support for diet and exercise programs by health insurance). *Emotional* and *encouraging* (appraisal) support are very similar. Emotional support involves encouragement and appreciation for the person affected and also sharing concerns. Encouraging support focuses on feedback and affirmation (Taiminen et al., 2020). However, social support is not synonymous with a network or ecosystem. The number of friends, membership in a sports club, the frequency of contact with a nutritionist should not be equated with social support, as an ecosystem is only a prerequisite for social support. For example, friends can also be a burden when those affected in the maintenance stage have to justify choosing a low-calorie dish when they go to a restaurant together. In addition, the number of friends says nothing about the quality of the support received.

To represent the maintenance stage from the perspective of those affected, the approach of the Customer Journey is chosen (Sect. 3.2). During the maintenance stage, those affected interact with people and organizations that offer support services or measures. The role and relevance of these interaction partners in maintaining a healthy lifestyle is examined using the ecosystem approach (Sect. 3.3).

3.2 The Customer Journey: A Tool for Visualizing the Maintenance Stage from the Perspective of Those Affected

The Customer Journey is adressed in the context of customer experience management and provides a structured and vivid representation of the experiences that customers have when purchasing a product or using a service (Stickdorn & Schneider, 2019). In the present context, it is about the experiences that those affected make in the phase of maintaining a healthy lifestyle. These include, for example, whether and where challenges arise, how they feel about it, and who they contact to overcome them. Customer Journey Mapping is a technique that enables professionals to better understand customer experiences. The following describes the elements of a customer journey, defines the concept of customer experience, and finally discusses the levels of a customer journey.

3.2.1 Elements of a Customer Journey and the Customer Experience

Based on a literature review, Bernard and Andritsos (2017) list components of Customer Journey Mapping, which are explained below: customer, journey, mapping, target orientation, touchpoint, timeline, channel, phase, customer experience, level, and multimedia.

The *customer*, whether female or male, is the stakeholder who purchases a product or uses a service. The purchase of a product or the use of a service is referred to as a *journey*, i.e., a typical path that a customer follows. A distinction is made between two types of journey: The expected journey is designed by internal stakeholders to describe what an ideal journey could look like. At the same time, it can also identify opportunities for new services. In contrast, the actual journey describes how it is experienced from the customer's perspective and what needs or problems arise when using the services. *Mapping* is a process that consists of tracking and describing the reactions and experiences of customers when using a service, describing and visualising them in a kind of map and documenting them. When mapping the customer journey, the *goal orientation* of the customers should be taken into account. Hamilton and Price (2019) point to the existence of overarching and subordinate goals. For example, the overarching goal of a customer journey could be to recover from an illness, which includes a customer journey with the subordinate goal of "getting medication". A customer journey consists of various *touchpoints*. A touchpoint is a point of contact where there is an interaction between the customer and the products or service offerings of service providers. A customer can go through the same touchpoints several times, but can also miss a planned touchpoint or end the journey unexpectedly. Lemon and Verhoef (2016) distinguish four categories of touchpoints:

1. *Brand-owned* touchpoints are designed and managed by the company. Their control is subject to the company. These include, for example, the website and the products or services offered.
2. *Partner-owned* touchpoints are customer interactions that are jointly designed and managed by the company and one or more partners, such as sales partners. Occasionally, the distinction between brand-owned and partner-owned touchpoints blurs, for example, when an app developed by a company that runs on Android and iOS is affected in its functionality by updates to the operating systems of Google and Apple.
3. *Customer-owned* touchpoints cannot be influenced or controlled by the company, its partners, or others. An example is a patient's exchange with her husband. Customer-owned touchpoints are particularly important and prevalent after purchase, when individual consumption and use take centre stage.
4. *Social, external* touchpoints, such as other customers, influences from peers, or independent sources of information, can also play an important role.

The *timeline* describes the duration of the journey from the first to the last touchpoint. By selecting the *channel*, the customer determines how the interaction with the touchpoints will take place, e.g., via an information desk or via social media. A customer journey consists of various *phases* (stages), which are referred to differently in the literature, e.g., "pre-purchase, purchase, and post-purchase situations" (Homburg et al., 2017, p. 384); "pre-core, core, and post-core service encounters" (Voorhees et al., 2017, p. 269) and "search, purchase, experience, and reflect" phases (Dellaert, 2019, p. 243).

Customer experiences are multidimensional constructs that encompass the cognitive, emotional, behavioral, sensory, and social responses of the customer to a company's offerings throughout the entire customer journey (Følstad & Kvale, 2018; Lemon & Verhoef, 2016). Just as there is a hierarchy of goals, different *levels* can be distinguished in customer journey mapping. On a higher level, overarching goals are pursued (for example, the journey "getting healthy" is depicted), while on the subordinate level, various journeys (for example, "getting medication") are described. With the help of *multimedia*, e.g., audio, video, photos, and sketches, the customer journey is visualized in an appealing way and can contribute to its understanding.

Becker et al. (2020) note that recently there have been calls for a customer-oriented view of the customer journey: Heinonen and Strandvik (2015) argue that for a better understanding of value creation processes, the focus should not be predominantly on how service providers involve their customers in their processes, but on how consumers interact with various actors in their lifeworld. According to Hamilton and Price (2019), true customer orientation requires an understanding of the respective customer journeys to achieve the big and small life goals. These demands emphasise the need to deal with the goals of consumers in customer journeys and not just with the purchase of products or services (Becker et al., 2020). A goal-oriented view of customer journeys can be particularly useful for service practice: it provides a holistic picture of the processes that customers go through on their way to the goal and of the possible interactions with various participants. This holistic view enables a company or organisation to better understand how its offering fits into these processes, how the individual customer journeys are connected with each other and which elements outside the direct control of the company influence the customer experience (Becker et al., 2020). A goal-oriented view of the customer journey offers companies the opportunity to develop convincing solutions (Epp & Price, 2011) and innovations (Patrício et al., 2011) that help their customers achieve their goals and ultimately increase their well-being.

3.2.2   Levels of a Customer Journey

The structuring of the customer journey into the three levels "Consumer-journey level", "Customer-journey level" and "Touchpoint level" (Becker et al., 2020) is adopted as the framework model for this study (see Fig. 3.1). This structuring takes into account the importance of goal orientation and acknowledges that there is a goal hierarchy.

At the level of the *Consumer Journey*, customers pursue overarching goals (e.g., maintaining a healthy lifestyle). A *Consumer Journey* includes several *Customer Journeys,* which are aimed at achieving subordinate goals (e.g., eating healthily, getting enough exercise). During the Customer Journeys, customers interact with different service providers and market participants (e.g., nutritionist, sports clubs). Pursuing a single

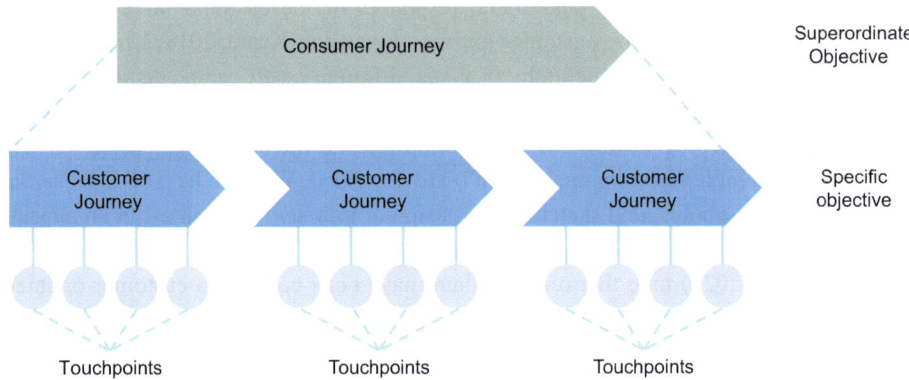

Fig. 3.1 Levels of a Customer Journey

Customer Journey can support the achievement of one or more subordinate goals, but it is not sufficient for an overarching goal achievement. For example, if someone exercises regularly but eats a very fat and carbohydrate-rich diet, maintaining a healthy lifestyle will not be successful. Each Customer Journey includes several touchpoints. At the "Touchpoint level", the achievement of a goal of a lower level of abstraction and thus a very specific task (e.g., 30 min. jogging) is in the focus.

When aiming to lead or maintain a healthy lifestyle, cognitive and behavior-related processes take place. Customers compare the actual situation, in which they find themselves due to their affective, cognitive, sensory, social, and physical experiences, with their goals (cognitive processes) and then act to achieve the respective goals or to minimize the discrepancy between the current and desired state (goal setting). This is by no means a linear and one-time process, rather this target/actual state takes place again and again. These are iterative processes that occur and customers also encounter obstacles and challenges. It is important to understand that the cognitive and behavior-related processes at the "Consumer-journey level", "Customer-journey level" and "Touchpoint level" take place simultaneously. When a customer interacts with a specific touchpoint to achieve a specific goal, this person is simultaneously undertaking a Consumer Journey to achieve an overarching goal (Becker et al., 2020).

3.3 Ecosystems: An Overview

The origin of the ecosystem view comes from biology. A natural ecosystem is a habitat in which different organisms coexist. Coexistence in such ecosystems is often characterized by collaboration as the most promising survival strategy (Farhadi, 2019). In his article *"Predators and Prey: A New Ecology of Competition"*, Moore, 1993 was the first to adapt the mechanisms of natural-biological ecosystems to business economics (Farhadi, 2019). In recent years, a large number of scientific publications have appeared on the term ecosystem, which have produced various ecosystem types and definitions (Jacobides et al., 2018).

Some typologies that describe the characteristics of ecosystems are explained below. The role of the actors varies between the different types of ecosystems. Table 3.1 provides an overview of various ecosystem definitions, whereby only those approaches being used that are relevant to the present study.

In all ecosystem types, value creation is fragmented and takes place in a network to which various actors with different abilities can connect (Adner, 2017; Faber et al., 2019; Jacobides et al., 2018; Vargo & Lusch, 2016). The service ecosystem perspective is relevant for the present study, because in order to pursue and maintain a healthy lifestyle, affected individuals use services from different service providers. The interaction of service providers with other actors in an ecosystem determines the value that is generated (Lusch et al., 2010). For example, if the health insurance company financially supports physical activities in a gym, this can have a positive effect on the motivation of

Table 3.1 Overview of ecosystem definitions

Term	Description
Service Ecosystem	A self-adapting system of actors who share resources and thereby pursue a common goal (Vargo & Lusch, 2016). A service is not provided by a single provider but rather individual parts of the service are combined by different parties to create an overall service that adds value and is difficult to imitate. (Leimeister, 2020).
Business Ecosystem	Can be described as a dynamically developing community of independent actors (companies and other stakeholders). The participants interact on the basis of harmonised technologies, standards, and rules (Burkhalter, 2019) in order to generate value-adding services and products for customers. The autonomous actors always pursue a common vision that that is aligned with their own vision (Adner, 2017).
Digital Business Ecosystem	Collaboration and knowledge transfer among the actors takes place exclusively via information and communication technologies. The term "Business Ecosystem" and the associated mechanisms of action remain unchanged (Corallo et al., 2007; Faber et al., 2019).

individual people and lead to them exercising more. However, this incentive does not have the same for everyone. For other peole affected who prefer to meet up with their friends for a weekly running session outdoors, this incentive is not effective. The example shows that the value and benefit of an ecosystem differ for the various actors and therefore needs to be determined individually. The value can include individual, social, technological, and cultural components (Leimeister, 2020). The Service Ecosystem perspective emphasizes that value is co-created within exchange systems with multiple actors. In these systems, common and lasting institutional arrangements—rules, roles, norms, and beliefs—determine resource integration and service exchange (Vargo & Lusch, 2016). It is not possible speak of a pure Digital Business Ecosystem. Nevertheless, in the exchange between the various actors in the health system information and communication technology (ICT) is playing an increasingly important role. Those affected use different apps that support them in setting nutrition and exercise goals and in monitoring these goals. Also, in the exchange with doctors, physiotherapists, or nutrition scientists, ICT is becoming increasingly important.

3.3.1   Characteristics of Ecosystems

Ecosystems are characterized by certain properties (Fuller et al., 2019):

1) Open and dynamic system with multilateral relationships
Every ecosystem consists of more than two actors who are involved in multilateral relationships with each other. In addition to private sector companies, these are government institutions, NGOs, consumers, and other stakeholders (Hileman et al., 2020). Each actor

maintains direct and indirect relationships not only with one, but with several actors. For example, a doctor recommends a diet change to a patient and refers her to a nutritionist. Ideally, the doctor and nutritionist communicate with each other. If the patient follows the advice of the nutritionist, she will change her food purchasing behavior and consume more fruits and vegetables. In addition to these information and goods flows, financial transactions also play a role. The patient pays a health insurance premium, and the doctor and nutritionist invoice their services to the health insurance company. The described network of relationships cannot be broken down into bilateral interactions, as the system only works as a whole (Adner, 2017). Since the system is open, actors can enter and leave at any time (Farhadi, 2019). For example, companies can enter that not only offer healthy recipe suggestions by means of an app, but also give patients the opportunity to monitor their calorie intake themselves or receive spontaneous help with nutritional questions via chat. In the medium to long term, only those supplying actors who can provide added value to the ecosystem will remain (Farhadi, 2019). For nutritionists, this may mean having to change their own range of services. Offering consultation hours via Zoom or telephone or setting up a chat funcion that satisfies the need for spontaneous patient inquiries without having to go to the practice can strengthen their position in the system. If this does not succeed, nutritionists risk losing customers and consequently having to give up their position in the ecosystem in the medium to long term. This reveals another characteristic of ecosystems: Although the participants generally collaborate with each other, they can also compete (Moore, 1996). This constellation is referred to as "coopetition" (Gnyawali & Park, 2011). For an ecosystem to continue to develop and innovate on an ongoing basis, an optimal mix of cooperation and competition is essential (Moore, 1996). For example, traditional nutritionists can compete with providers of app-based nutrition programs, but at the same time collaborate in other areas (e.g., joint lobbying for reimbursement of services by insurance companies).

2) Modularity and Complementarity
Ecosystems are complementary systems characterized by mutually complementary elements, allowing for the provision of modular services. A service, consisting of interdependent components, can be provided cost-effectively and efficiently by various participants in a consortium (Jacobides et al., 2018). Applied to the health ecosystem, this could look as follows: A doctor prescribes a diabetes patient in addition to a diet change a medication, which the patient obtains from the pharmacy. The pharmacist not only advises the patient on correct dosage, but also replaces the prescribed medication with an equivalent, but cheaper generic. In the ecosystem, this service provision takes place in a network consortium. As part of modularity, all those involved focus on their competencies. In addition to competence aspects, other aspects (e.g., cost aspects) must also be considered. Specifically, the question arises as to which services a patient visits a doctor. Certain health counseling services can be provided more cost-effectively by pharmacies. In addition, patients have the advantage that appointments for e.g., blood pressure measurements in the pharmacy are usually not necessary or can be made more

quickly at a pharmacy, thus increasing the overall perceived service quality from the patient's perspective. The question of who provides which services in the healthcare system and which interests play a role in this is analysed in more detail in Sect. 3.3.2. In addition to modularity, complementarity is a particular characteristic of ecosystems. Complementarity means that the individual ecosystem elements (activities, competencies or resources of the actors) combine so advantageously that the existence of one element increases the value of the other. Consequently, the value of the ecosystem is always greater than the sum of the individual elements (Lechner & Dexheimer, 2019). In the aforementioned example, the pharmacist's consulting service can be considered complementary. By using an equivalent, but cheaper medication, lower costs are charged to the insurance. This contributes to cost containment in the health system.

3) Altered Value Creation Logic

Ecosystems are characterized by a modified value creation logic (Jacobides et al., 2018), in which consumers play a central role. While they were long considered passive, they are now actively involved in service provision in ecosystems (Payne et al., 2008). The active role of patients is also emphasized in the context of healthcare ecosystems. In the sense of co-creation, patients, for example, provide their own data, from which personalized services and products can be created. They also take over activities from the service provider side (here from the doctor or the pharmacy), for example, when they monitor their blood sugar levels using digital tools. Consequently, consumers also contribute to the value enhancement of an ecosystem.

3.3.2   Roles in Ecosystems

An ecosystem consists of several actors who assume certain roles. Due to environmental dynamics, determining the boundaries of an ecosystem and thus also the participants in the ecosystem is difficult. However, the actors always assume a certain role (Moore, 1993). Moore (1993) primarily focused on those participants who assume a leadership role in the ecosystem (Leaders). Most role concepts take a strategy-oriented perspective and define the roles either by the particular behavior associated with them (e.g., Dominator or Opportunist), by a specific functional contribution (e.g., Regulator, Sponsor), or by a specific characteristic related to the actor (e.g., Entrepreneur, Landlord). Consequently, these roles remain detached from a specific value purpose (in this case, maintaining a healthy lifestyle), which forms the anchor point around which an ecosystem develops (Burkhalter, 2019). From an SDL perspective (see Sect. 3.1), Voima et al. (2011) offer an interesting starting point by emphasizing that roles can be defined in relation to a service (materialized common purpose). Accordingly, four role archetypes that are related to each other in an ecosystem can be defined (Burkhalter, 2019):

Service Users are actors who achieve their individual goals through the utilization of the service. So, when actors assume the user role, they use their own resources to benefit from the service result.

Service Providers are actors who achieve individual goals by providing offers neces-sary for service provision. When actors assume the provider role, they undertake activi-ties to use their own resources and indirectly benefit from the service result (e.g., through monetary compensation or social compensation, such as status or reputation).

The Service Orchestrator is an actor who achieves individual goals by coordinating activities and associated resources. When actors assume the role of the service orchestra-tor, they use resources from this role to indirectly benefit from the service result, either through compensation from the user or the provider. This can be a monetary or non-mon-etary compensation.

Service Contributors are actors who achieve individual goals by supporting the users, providers, or orchestrators in their specific functions. When actors assume the role of the contributor, they use resources to indirectly benefit from the service result. Contribu-tors receive compensation through a monetary or non-monetary reward from the user, the providers, or from the orchestrators.

Each role archetype is characterized by unique abilities in relation to a specific ser-vice. This means that the abilities of a role archetype can only fully unfold in interaction with the other role archetypes and that the abilities of the various archetypes that make up the ecosystem can overlap (Burkhalter, 2019).

Each role can be assumed by single or multiple legally independent actors who are socially and economically interconnected. The actors pursue common objectives based on explicitly formulated or latent needs. They use their operand and operant resources to contribute to the service result. The result of this commitment, consisting of monetary and non-monetary benefits and risks (costs), is balanced by each participant with their individual goals. Only when actors recognize a balance between the associated benefits and perceived costs in their respective roles are they willing to participate in a particu-lar ecosystem in the long term (Burkhalter, 2019). The orchestrator plays a particularly important role in the ecosystem in understanding and eighing up the needs, but also in guiding and balancing the resource use of the respective actors. This role should ensure that the actors maximise their contribution to achieve the common goal.

3.4   Health Economics and Interprofessionalism

Health economics, at the intersection of health and economic sciences, primarily deals with cost-benefit considerations against the backdrop of increasingly cost-intensive medical care systems in the Western world (Breyer et al., 2013; Van der Beek & Van der Beek, 2012). In almost all countries, the proportion of the gross domestic product (GDP) spent on health continues to rise (Federal Statistical Office, 2021; Lago-Peñas et al., 2013). Since health costs in virtually all countries have risen more than wages over the last 100 years (Breyer et al., 2013), the pressure for efficiency on the healthcare system has also steadily increased. Economic considerations in dealing with the limited health budget are gaining importance over purely medically indicated treatment decisions, which do not or only partially consider cost-benefit factors. Efficiency considerations also increasingly play a role in the official assessment of services of the compulsory health insurance. For example, Swiss legislation requires that services at the expense of the compulsory basic insurance must meet the criteria effectiveness, appropriateness and cost-efficiency (FOPH, 2011). Thus, services must not only be medically effective, but also economically justifiable.

Health economics assumes a fundamentally rational individual who weighs the respective advantages and disadvantages when making any decision between options (Braun & Gautschi, 2011). However, so-called information asymmetries in health economics must be taken into account (Simon, 1959), as there is often a large knowledge gap between professionals and patients. Thus, a patient often lacks the knowledge to rationally choose between different medical treatment options (Breyer et al., 2013). Therefore, professionals have a higher decision-making power compared to other markets. The complete information of the consumer required by economic sciences for a rational decision is often not given in the healthcare system. Therefore, the analysis of the incentives that affect the providers in the healthcare system is important, as their design significantly shapes the treatment decisions.

In addition, the healthcare system in almost all countries is a heavily regulated, or (partially) state market, in which free competition between provider and consumer does not play a role (Pitschas, 1999). For example, in almost all Western countries, patients only partially bear the direct costs of their consumption of health services, another part is covered by a (state) insurance, which is designed differently depending on the country (OECD, 2021; Zawada et al., 2017). Government interventions in the health market also influence individual consumption decisions.

In many Western countries, the health insurance systems are strongly curative-oriented: The insurance benefits mainly relate to the coverage of disease-related costs. (Primary) prevention, i.e. the attempt to avoid future disease costs, is often much less or not at all covered by the corresponding state insurances (Wang, 2018). For example, subscriptions to fitness studios, participation in regular sports training or nutritional coaching in the Swiss healthcare system are not paid for by the basic insurance. Some, chargeable supplementary insurances partially pay a subsidy for such programs, but such supplementary insurances are voluntary and are not available to all persons (e.g. those with risk factors). Accordingly, there is only a small incentive for preventive measures (such as weight reduction) on both the provider and consumer side in the healthcare system, if the disease costs caused by overweight are later covered by an insurance.

Regarding the individual's decision-making basis for or against health-promoting behavior (or its maintenance), it can therefore be assumed that short-term benefit considerations often speak against health-promoting behavior. The immediate benefit gain from consuming a chocolate bar is opposed to the very abstract long-term risk of disease.

In sum, this individual, rational behavior leads to the so-called prevention paradox: Preventive behavior brings a lot to the entire society by avoiding individual severe diseases, but little to the individual and vice versa (Franzkowiak, 2018). An individually short-term health-damaging behavior is thus per se economically explainable and it requires suitable incentives, tools and information to influence the corresponding individual cost-benefit considerations.

The incentives for the involved professions are also well studied from a health economics perspective. With today's remuneration system, which in many countries relies on ex-post payment for individual services, there is little incentive for prevention or cost-damping measures (Felder et al., 2017; Kaiser et al., 2019). By not involving service providers in the "success" of the treatment, but on the contrary even profiting financially from diseases, corresponding false incentives are created (Felder et al., 2019). For example, if a patient is well advised preventively about nutrition, she will subsequently make little use of health services for diseases that can be traced back to an unhealthy diet. She is, so to speak, lost as a customer. However, if someone struggles with the consequences of an unhealthy diet for a long time, he or she will have to use health services again and again.

From a societal perspective, a system would be desirable that sets incentives for the prevention of diseases and allows service providers to work together in an ideal and cost-efficient way. This is summarized under the term interprofessionalism, which can be defined as close coordination and agreement of professionals from different disciplines and professions (Sottas et al., 2016). Today, many health systems suffer from the fact that they do not set incentives for cooperation and coordination of professionals due to the remuneration scheme with individual service tariffs (Felder et al., 2019). Since each profession is compensated for its specific service, but cooperative services are often not or only insufficiently represented in the remuneration scheme, cooperation is not promoted (Gurtner & Wettstein, 2019). In addition, there are deficits in education and training, which is strongly profession-specific and also hinders cooperation between the various providers in the health care system (Bianchi et al., 2019; Huber et al., 2020).

On the other hand, research on interprofessionalism shows that successful cooperation and coordination of providers in the health care system can potentially save costs or at least achieve a higher quality of care at the same costs (Liesch et al., 2020). The coordination itself is associated with some effort, but this is at least compensated by the gains of a better treatment thanks to the corresponding cooperation. For example, it may be worthwhile for a person with obesity to clarify interprofessionally at an early stage which health professionals should carry out which intervention when and how these interventions are coordinated and their successes measured. If there is no corresponding cooperation, a "run through the institutions" may ensue, in which the patient receives contradictory instructions from different health professionals, which can significantly reduce motivation and is not conducive to the course of the disease.

A specific focus of the health economic consideration lies in the question of which profession is best suited for which service. Western health systems tend to be strongly doctor-centered. However, these are usually the most expensive health service providers. From a health economic perspective, it is therefore necessary to ask whether various medical services can be transferred to professions that work more cost-effectively

(Schmelzer et al., 2020). If pharmacies, dieticians or prevention experts can take over medical services, this so-called task-shift between health professions leads to lower costs for society as a whole.

3.5   Conclusion and Relevance for the Present Research Project

From the perspective of service management and health economics, the present research project can be assigned to Transformative Service Research (TSR). If those affected manage to transform their lifestyle sustainably, their quality of life is increasing. To answer the question of how the maintenance stage is designed from the perspective of those affected, the instrument of the Customer Journey is used. Chapter 7 summarizes the empirical results of the present research project and explains using the results from 20 in-depth interviews how the customer journey is specifically organised in the maintenance phase. Here, the micro level of Transformative Service Research is addressed.

To clarify the roles of those affected and the other actors, the ecosystem perspective is adopted. This is where interprofessionalism comes into play. Interprofessional collaboration exists when two or more members of different professional groups in the health care system work hand in hand and make decisions together to solve problems or provide services. In addition to the micro level, the meso and macro level of TSR is at the center of attention. The empirical results are summarized in Chapts. 7 and 8.

Finally, the toolbox presented in Chap. 10, which summarizes the project's recommendations for action, builds on the basics presented in Chap. 3 and thus contributes to the further development of the current state of research.

References

Adner, R. (2017). Ecosystem as structure: An actionable construct for strategy. *Journal of Management, 43*(1), 39–58. https://doi.org/10.1177/0149206316678451.

Anderson, L., Ostrom, A. L., & Bitner, M. J. (2011). *Surrounded by services: A new lens for examining the influence of services as social structures on well-being.* Working Study, WP Carey School of Business, Arizona State University.

BAG. (2011). *Operationalisierung der Begriffe Wirksamkeit, Zweckmässigkeit und Wirtschaftlichkeit, Arbeitspapier, Version 2.0.* https://www.bag.admin.ch/dam/bag/de/dokumente/kuv-leistungen/bezeichnung-der-leistungen/AntragsprozesseAllgemeine Leistungen/operationalisierung-der-begriffe-wzw-arbeitspapier-vom-21-07-2011.pdf.download.pdf/Operationalisierung der Begriffe WZW Arbeitspapier vom 21.07.2011.pdf..

Ballantine, P. W., & Stephenson, R. J. (2011). Help me, I'm fat! Social support in online weight loss networks. *Journal of Consumer Behaviour, 10*(6), 332–337. https://doi.org/10.1002/cb.374.

Becker, L., Jaakkola, E., & Halinen, A. (2020). Toward a goal-oriented view of customer journeys. *Journal of Service Management, 31*(4), 767–790. https://doi.org/10.1108/JOSM-11-2019-0329.

Bernard, G., & Andritsos, P. (2017). A process mining based model for customer journey mapping. In Forum and doctoral consortium papers presented at the 29th International Conference on Advanced Information Systems Engineering (CAiSE 2017). *CEUR Workshop Proceedings* (Vol. 1848, pp. 49–56).

Bianchi, M., Meli, G., Caitata Zufferey, M., Di Giulio, P., & Pedrazzani, C. (2019). *Le potentiel de la formation interprofessionnelle de base dans le domaine de la santé suisse: Analyse de l'impact d'une expérience de formation interprofessionnelle en Suisse italienne. Rapport à l'attention de l'Office fédéral de la santé publique (OFSP).* SUPSI.

Braun, N., & Gautschi, T. (2011). *Rational-Choice-Theorie.* Juventa.

Breyer, F., Zweifel, P., & Kifmann, M. (2013). *Gesundheitsökonomik* (6., vollst. erw. und überarb. Aufl.). Springer Gabler. https://doi.org/10.1007/978-3-642-30894-9.

Bundesamt für Statistik. (2021). *Ausgaben für das Gesundheitswesen.* https://www.bfs.admin.ch/bfs/de/home/statistiken/querschnittsthemen/wohlfahrtsmessung/alle-indikatoren/gesellschaft/gesundheitsausgaben.html.

Burkhalter, M. (2019). *Allocentric Business Models – An Allocentric Business Model Ontology for the Orchestration of Value Co-Creation using the Example of Financial Service Ecosystems* [University of St. Gallen]. https://www.e-helvetica.nb.admin.ch/api/download/urn%3Anbn%3Ach%3Abel-1496943%3ADis4940.pdf/Dis4940.pdf.

Chan, K. W., Yim, C. K., & Lam, S. S. K. (2010). Is customer participation in value creation a double-edged sword? Evidence from professional financial services across cultures. *Journal of Marketing, 74*(3), 48–64. https://doi.org/10.1509/jmkg.74.3.48.

Chandler, J. D., & Lusch, R. F. (2015). Service systems: A broadened framework and research agenda on value propositions, engagement, and service experience. *Journal of Service Research, 18*(1), 6–22. https://doi.org/10.1177/1094670514537709.

Corallo, A., Passiante, G., & Prencipe, A. (Eds.). (2007). *The digital business ecosystem.* Edward.

Dellaert, B. G. C. (2019). The consumer production journey: Marketing to consumers as co-producers in the sharing economy. *Journal of the Academy of Marketing Science, 47*(2), 238–254. https://doi.org/10.1007/s11747-018-0607-4.

Dellande, S., Gilly, M. C., & Graham, J. L. (2004). Gaining compliance and losing weight: The role of the service provider in health care services. *Journal of Marketing, 68*(3), 78–91. https://doi.org/10.1509/jmkg.68.3.78.34764.

Epp, A. M., & Price, L. L. (2011). Designing solutions around customer network identity goals. *Journal of Marketing, 75*(2), 36–54. https://doi.org/10.1509/jm.75.2.36.

Faber, A., Riemhofer, M., Rehm, S.-V., & Bondel, G. (2019). *A systematic mapping study on business ecosystem types.* AMCIS.

Farhadi, N. (2019). Grundlagen: Gemeinsam stärker sein. In N. Farhadi (Eds.), *Cross-Industry Ecosystems: Grundlagen, Archetypen, Modelle und strategische Ansätze* (S. 5–22). Springer Fachmedien Wiesbaden. https://doi.org/10.1007/978-3-658-26129-0_2

Felder, S., Meyer, S., Merki, M., & Plaza, C. (2017). *Komplexpauschalen in der Schweiz: Umsetzbarkeit integraler Vergütungssysteme im Schweizer Gesundheitswesen.* [Gutachten im Auftrag des Bundesamtes für Gesundheit BAG]. Institut für Wirtschaftsstudien Basel.

Felder, S., Meyer, S., Merki, M., Plaza, C., Poledna, T., & Rosemann, T. (2019). *Komplexpauschalen in der Schweiz: Umsetzbarkeit integraler Vergütungssysteme im Schweizer Gesundheitswesen.* [Gutachten im Auftrag des Bundesamtes für Gesundheit BAG]. Institut für Wirtschaftsstudien Basel.

Følstad, A., & Kvale, K. (2018). Customer journeys: A systematic literature review. *Journal of Service Theory and Practice, 28*(2), 196–227. https://doi.org/10.1108/JSTP-11-2014-0261.

Franzkowiak, P. (2018). Präventionsparadox. *Leitbegriffe der Gesundheitsförderung und Prävention: Glossar zu Konzepten, Strategien und Methoden.* Bundeszentrale für gesundheitliche Aufklärung. https://doi.org/10.17623/BZGA:224-I094-2.0.

Fuller, J., Jacobides, M., & Reeves, M. (2019). The myths and realities of business ecosystems. *MIT Sloan Management Review, 60*(3), 1–9.

Gnyawali, D. R., & Park, B.-J. (Robert). (2011). Co-opetition between giants: Collaboration with competitors for technological innovation. *Research Policy, 40*(5), 650–663. https://doi.org/10.1016/j.respol.2011.01.009.

Gurtner, S., & Wettstein, M. (2019). *Interprofessionelle Zusammenarbeit im Gesundheitswesen—Anreize und Hindernisse in der Berufsausübung.* Berner Fachhochschule – Wirtschaft, Institut Unternehmensentwicklung.

Hamilton, R., & Price, L. L. (2019). Consumer journeys: Developing consumer-based strategy. *Journal of the Academy of Marketing Science, 47*(2), 187–191. https://doi.org/10.1007/s11747-019-00636-y.

Heinonen, K., & Strandvik, T. (2015). Customer-dominant logic: Foundations and implications. *Journal of Services Marketing, 29*(6/7), 472–484. https://doi.org/10.1108/JSM-02-2015-0096.

Hileman, J., Kallstenius, I., Häyhä, T., Palm, C., & Cornell, S. (2020). Keystone actors do not act alone: A business ecosystem perspective on sustainability in the global clothing industry. *PLoS ONE, 15*(10), e0241453. https://doi.org/10.1371/journal.pone.0241453.

Homburg, C., Jozić, D., & Kuehnl, C. (2017). Customer experience management: Toward implementing an evolving marketing concept. *Journal of the Academy of Marketing Science, 45*(3), 377–401. https://doi.org/10.1007/s11747-015-0460-7.

House, J. S. (1981). *Work stress and social support.* Addison-Wesley.

Huber, M., Spiegel-Steinmann, B., Schwärzler, P., Kerry-Krause, M. J., Kaap-Fröhlich, S., Panfil, E.-M., Witt, C., Feusi, E., Gerber-Grote, A., & Melloh, M. (2020). *Kompetenzen zur interprofessionellen Zusammenarbeit und geeignete Unterrichtsformate.* Bern: Bundesamt für Gesundheit. https://digitalcollection.zhaw.ch/handle/11475/19186

Hwang, K. O., Ottenbacher, A. J., Green, A. P., Cannon-Diehl, M. R., Richardson, O., Bernstam, E. V., & Thomas, E. J. (2010). Social support in an Internet weight loss community. *International Journal of Medical Informatics, 79*(1), 5–13. https://doi.org/10.1016/j.ijmedinf.2009.10.003

Jacobides, M. G., Cennamo, C., & Gawer, A. (2018). Towards a theory of ecosystems. *Strategic Management Journal, 39*(8), 2255–2276. https://doi.org/10.1002/smj.2904.

Kaiser, N., Amann, F., Meier, N., Inderbitzi, L., Haering, B., Eicher, M., & Stanic, J. (2019). *Berufsausübung: Potenziale für Interprofessionalität.* [Schlussbericht Mandat 4 im Auftrag des Förderprogramms Interprofessionalität des Bundesamts für Gesundheit.]. Bern: Bundesamt für Gesundheit.

Kuppelwieser, V. G., & Finsterwalder, J. (2016). Transformative service research and service dominant logic: Quo Vaditis? *Journal of Retailing and Consumer Services, 28,* 91–98. https://doi.org/10.1016/j.jretconser.2015.08.011.

Lago-Peñas, S., Cantarero-Prieto, D., & Blázquez-Fernández, C. (2013). On the relationship between GDP and health care expenditure: A new look. *Economic Modelling, 32,* 124–129. https://doi.org/10.1016/j.econmod.2013.01.021

Lechner, C., & Dexheimer, M. J. (2019). Eine neue Strategie im digitalen Zeitalter? *OrganisationsEntwicklung, 3,* 38–43.

Leimeister, J. M. (2020). *Dienstleistungsengineering und -management: Data-driven service innovation* (2., vollständig aktualisierte und erweiterte Aufl.). Springer Gabler. https://doi.org/10.1007/978-3-662-59858-0.

Lemon, K. N., & Verhoef, P. C. (2016). Understanding customer experience throughout the customer journey. *Journal of Marketing, 80*(6), 69–96. https://doi.org/10.1509/jm.15.0420.

Liesch, R., Berchtold, P., & Künzi, K. (2020). *Kosten-Nutzen-Analyse interprofessioneller Zusammenarbeit. Empirische Analyse am Beispiel stationärer Klinken der Inneren Medizin und der Psychiatrie*. Büro für arbeits-und sozialpolitische Studien BASS/College für Management im Gesundheitswesen.

Lusch, R. F., Vargo, S. L., & Tanniru, M. (2010). Service, value networks and learning. *Journal of the Academy of Marketing Science, 38*(1), 19–31. https://doi.org/10.1007/s11747-008-0131-z.

Montani, J.-P., Schutz, Y., & Dulloo, A. G. (2015). Dieting and weight cycling as risk factors for cardiometabolic diseases: Who is really at risk?: Weight cycling and cardiometabolic risks. *Obesity Reviews, 16*, 7–18. https://doi.org/10.1111/obr.12251.

Moore, J. F. (1993). Predators and prey: A new ecology of competition. *Harvard Business Review.* https://hbr.org/1993/05/predators-and-prey-a-new-ecology-of-competition.

Moore, J. F. (1996). *The death of competition: Leadership and strategy in the age of business ecosystems*. Harper Collins.

OECD. (2021). *Health spending*. OECD. http://data.oecd.org/healthres/health-spending.htm.

Osterwalder, A., Pigneur, Y., Bernardakēs, G. N., Smith, A., & Papadakos, T. (2015). *Value proposition design: Entwickeln Sie Produkte und Services, die Ihre Kunden wirklich wollen*. Campus.

Parkinson, J., Schuster, L., Mulcahy, R., & Taiminen, H. M. (2017). Online support for vulnerable consumers: A safe place? *Journal of Services Marketing, 31*(4/5), 412–422. https://doi.org/10.1108/JSM-05-2016-0197.

Patrício, L., Fisk, R. P., Falcão e Cunha, J., & Constantine, L. (2011). Multilevel service design: From customer value constellation to service experience blueprinting. *Journal of Service Research, 14*(2), 180–200. https://doi.org/10.1177/1094670511401901.

Payne, A. F., Storbacka, K., & Frow, P. (2008). Managing the co-creation of value. *Journal of the Academy of Marketing Science, 36*(1), 83–96. https://doi.org/10.1007/s11747-007-0070-0,

Pitschas, R. (1999). Gesundheitswesen zwischen Staat und Markt. In H. Häfner (Eds.), *Gesundheit—Unser höchstes Gut?* (S. 169–203). Springer. https://doi.org/10.1007/978-3-642-60166-8_9.

Previte, J., & Robertson, N. (2019). A continuum of transformative service exchange: Insights for service and social marketers. *Journal of Services Marketing, 33*(6), 671–686. https://doi.org/10.1108/JSM-10-2018-0280.

Schmelzer, S., Hollenstein, E., Stahl, J., Wirz, M., Huber, M., Nast, I., & Liberatore, F. (2020). *Task Shifting in der inter-professionellen Zusammenarbeit*. Winterthur: ZHAW Zürcher Hochschule für Angewandte Wissenschaften. https://doi.org/10.21256/zhaw-20950

Simon, H. A. (1959). Theories of decision-making in economics and behavioral science. *The American Economic Review, 49*, 3.

Sottas, B., Kissmann, S., & Brügger, S. (2016). *Interprofessionelle Ausbildung (IPE): Erfolgsfaktoren–Messinstrument–Best Practice Beispiele*. Sottas formative works.

Stickdorn, M., & Schneider, J. (Eds.). (2019). *This is service design thinking: Basics, tools, cases* (Paperback edition, 8th printing). BIS Publishers.

Taiminen, H., Taiminen, K., & Munnukka, J. (2020). Enabling transformative value creation through online weight loss services. *Journal of Services Marketing, 34*(6), 797–808. https://doi.org/10.1108/JSM-05-2019-0191.

Van der Beek, K., & Van der Beek, G. (2012). *Gesundheitsökonomik*. Wissenschaftsverlag.

Vargo, S. L., & Lusch, R. F. (2004). Evolving to a new dominant logic for marketing. *Journal of Marketing, 68*(1), 1–17. https://doi.org/10.1509/jmkg.68.1.1.24036.

Vargo, S. L., & Lusch, R. F. (2008). Service-dominant logic: Continuing the evolution. *Journal of the Academy of Marketing Science, 36*(1), 1–10. https://doi.org/10.1007/s11747-007-0069-6.

Vargo, S. L., & Lusch, R. F. (2016). Institutions and axioms: An extension and update of service-dominant logic. *Journal of the Academy of Marketing Science, 44*(1), 5–23. https://doi.org/10.1007/s11747-015-0456-3.

Voima, P., Heinonen, K., Strandvik, T., Mickelsson, K.-J., & Arantola-Hattab, J. (2011). A customer ecosystem perspective on service. *QUIS 12: Advances in Service Quality, Innovation and Excellence,* 1015–1024.

Voorhees, C. M., Fombelle, P. W., Gregoire, Y., Bone, S., Gustafsson, A., Sousa, R., & Walkowiak, T. (2017). Service encounters, experiences and the customer journey: Defining the field and a call to expand our lens. *Journal of Business Research, 79,* 269–280. https://doi.org/10.1016/j.jbusres.2017.04.014.

Wang, F. (2018). The roles of preventive and curative health care in economic development. *PLoS ONE, 13*(11), e0206808. https://doi.org/10.1371/journal.pone.0206808.

Zawada, A., Kolasa, K., Kronborg, C., Rabczenko, D., Rybnik, T., Lauridsen, J. T., Ceglowska, U., & Hermanowski, T. (2017). A comparison of the burden of out-of-pocket health payments in Denmark, Germany and Poland. *Global Policy, 8,* 123–130. https://doi.org/10.1111/1758-5899.12331.

Part II
Empirical Studies

Practical Measures for a Sustainable Lifestyle Change

4

Contents

Abstract

A central concern of behavior change is the identification of practical behavior change techniques from the fields of nutrition, exercise, and health, which contribute to the maintenance of a sustainable lifestyle. To determine these, three sub-studies were conducted: firstly, qualitative, guideline-based interviews with experts from the health sector, and secondly, interviews with those affected themselves. Thirdly, based on the interviews, prototypes for concrete, practical measures for sustainable lifestyle

© The Author(s), under exclusive license to Springer-Verlag GmbH, DE, part of Springer Nature 2024
A. Schäfer et al., *Maintaining a Healthy Lifestyle*,
https://doi.org/10.1007/978-3-662-69460-2_4

change were developed in a Design Thinking workshop with representatives from the health ecosystem. These include "goal setting and monitoring", "reward", "challenge sprints", "sponsor system", and "emergency button" and serve as the basis for the later impact study.

4.1   Determination of Sustainable Measures

The first study within the conducted project aims to answer the overarching research question: Which measures successfully support affected individuals in a sustainable lifestyle change? As outlined in Sect. 2.2, a measure in this case is understood as the concrete implementation of a behavior change technique (BCT). The scientific literature offers a wide range of behavior change techniques that help individuals change their lifestyle. Although it can be assumed that some of these behavior change techniques are also beneficial for the maintenance phase, there is currently no solid scientific evidence for this. Furthermore, the question needs to be answered as to how behavior change techniques can be designed as concrete measures to contribute to a sustainable lifestyle change. To close this research gap, three sub-studies were conducted with different methodological approaches and separate subordinate research questions:

1. Six qualitative, guideline-based interviews with experts from the health sector to answer the question: Which behavior change techniques are used in the treatment of individuals with diagnoses such as obesity and type 2 diabetes in the phase of maintaining a healthy lifestyle and which behavior change techniques prove to be successful?
2. Seven qualitative, guideline-based interviews with affected individuals to answer the question: Which of the identified behavior change techniques contribute to a sustainable lifestyle change from the perspective of those affected?
3. A Design Thinking Workshop with employees of service companies from the health sector to answer the question: How can the identified behavior change techniques be specifically designed as practical measures to support a sustainable lifestyle change?

The three sub-studies including the answers to the corresponding research questions are presented in the following Sect. 4.2 to 4.4. Section 4.5 summarizes the findings of the three sub-studies in a brief conclusion and answers the overarching research question.

4.2   Sub-study 1: Identification of Successful Behavior Change Techniques from the Perspective of Service Providers

Answer to research question 1: Which behavior change techniques are used in the treatment of individuals with diagnoses such as obesity and type 2 diabetes in the phase of maintaining a healthy lifestyle and prove to be successful?

4.2.1 Survey of Experts from the Health Sector

To identify successfully used behavior change techniques, six structured guideline-based interviews were conducted with professionals from the fields of medicine, nutrition, and physical activity. In the health ecosystem, these individuals play the role of providers and supporters. The goal of the interviews was to identify 1) effective behavior change techniques during the maintenance phase, 2) challenges, and 3) other influencing factors in the everyday life of those affected. Furthermore, it was discussed how the quality of the service product of a "comprehensive support service for maintaining a healthy lifestyle" can be designed through the interaction of the various ecosystem partners so that it has the most sustainable effect and offers assistance in everyday life for those affected. Finally, a validation of the effective interventions for the maintenance phase, as compiled from the literature (see Chap. 2), was undertaken. Using selective sampling (Przyborski & Wohlrab-Sahr, 2021), two doctors, two nutritionists, a diabetes counselor, and a physiotherapist from German-speaking Switzerland were selected for the discussions. Their experience in accompanying individuals with the diagnoses of obesity and type 2 diabetes was the decisive selection criterion.

For the identification of effective behavior change techniques in the maintenance phase, the interviewees based their responses on actual counseling processes of successful and failed individuals from their professional everyday life. This was followed by the identification of general influencing factors on the sustainability of measures as well as relevant and desirable interfaces within the health ecosystem. The approximately 60-minute interviews were recorded and transcribed in a meaningful way, so that a comparative topic analysis (Froschauer & Lueger, 2020) could be carried out after all interviews were completed.

4.2.2 Central Findings from the Perspective of Experts

The discussions provided a good insight into tested interventions, challenges of and influencing factors on those affected, as well as the interplay of ecosystem partners. The specific measures mentioned were linked with quotes from the interviews with the behavior change techniques mentioned in the literature. This enabled the identification of which techniques were significant for those affected across the various fields of activity of the respondents. The respondents repeatedly emphasized the inclusion of the social environment as a particularly successful behavior change technique, e.g. in connection with nutrition within a household or through joint exercise with a known person or in a group. Above all, the emotional and encouraging dimension of support was mentioned, for example by the partner who supports those affected through a joint change in diet. From the perspective of experts, interventions prove to be more promising if they are tailored individually to the needs of those affected. This refers in particular to setting goals that do not overwhelm those affected, but should be formulated in small steps as realistically achievable intermediate goals. Such achieved successes have a positive effect on the joy of the action carried out and thus on the autonomous motivation of those affected. According to the Self-Determination Theory by Deci and Ryan (2000), this has positive effects on maintaining a behavior change.

As challenges that those affected struggle with in the maintenance phase of their lifestyle change, experts named everyday stress, incisive experiences such as a separation or further illnesses, which make the situation of those affected more difficult. In addition, the educational level and social status of those affected could be identified as influencing factors on the success of lifestyle adjustment.

Regarding the interplay of ecosystem partners, the respondents attributed a positive effect on the sustainable impact of measures to close cooperation between the doctor and nutritionists. Through this cooperation, for example, goals can be set together and progress can be checked. Additional networking to exercise offers was described as desirable, as the pursuit of coordinated goals from the areas of nutrition and exercise is perceived as particularly promising. This is in line with the findings presented in Chap. 3 on the importance of health ecosystems, which were also considered valuable by the respondents.

Following the interviews, the described findings were compared with the successful behavior change techniques known from the literature and presented in Sect. 2.3. Due to the small sample of respondents, the findings of the broadly supported scientific study "Diabetes Prevention Program" (DPP) were additionally used for this purpose. The DPP aims to change lifestyle through a combination of calorie reduction measures, increasing physical activity, and accompanying lifestyle coaching. The results of the study show that participants achieved a decrease of 5 to 7 % of their body weight and reduced the risk of developing type 2 diabetes by 58 %. A follow-up study showed that ten years later, participants were still a third less likely to develop type 2 diabetes than people in a control group, thus proving the sustainable success of these combinations of measures (The Diabetes Prevention Program Research Group, 2002).

The findings from the literature and the interviews were presented to the business partners involved in the research project, checked by them for their practical relevance, and prioritized. This resulted in the following selection of behavior change techniques as the basis for the sub-study 2: "Goal Setting and Planning", "Feedback and Monitoring" as well as "Repetition and Substitution". A detailed description of these behavior change techniques can be found in Sect. 2.2.2.

4.3   Sub-study 2: Identification of Successful Behavior Change Techniques from the Perspective of Those Affected

Answer to research question 2: Which of the identified behavior change techniques contribute to a sustainable lifestyle change from the perspective of those affected?

4.3.1   Survey of Affected Individuals in the Maintenance Stage

Based on the presented findings, guideline-based interviews were conducted with seven individuals affected by the diagnoses of overweight and type 2 diabetes. The aim of the interviews was to validate the relevance of the behavior change techniques defined as priority for a sustainable lifestyle change. This was achieved by querying specific behavioral practices from the everyday life of the affected individuals.

The interviewed individuals were four men and three women from German-speaking Switzerland, aged between 34 and 63 years, who could be recruited for participation in the study through selective sampling. In some cases, contacts of the interviewed doctors as well as customers of Uplyfe, the health program provider involved in the project for lifestyle change, were used. The life circumstances in terms of employment, marital status, social position, and living situation of the interviewees were very different. However, what the interviewees had in common was that they had changed their lifestyle for health reasons more than four months before the interview and were thus in the maintenance phase of their lifestyle change.

The interviews were divided into three thematic blocks, starting with sociodemographic characteristics of the interviewees, followed by questions about the relevance of health ecosystem providers for maintaining a healthy lifestyle, and finally questions about specific measures for its maintenance.

As visual support, cards with icons of typical measures were used during the interview. When a service provider or a measure was mentioned, the corresponding card was laid out by the interviewer. Unexpected additional mentions by the interviewees were noted on blank cards, so that a collection of all mentioned service providers and measures emerged during the interviews. To ensure that no mentions were forgotten by the interviewees, the interviewers subsequently asked about further, previously unmentioned measures and health providers using the remaining prepared cards.

The interviews were recorded and transcribed, and the visual aids were photographed. The deductive coding of the interviews was done with the software MAXQDA (Mayring, 2015). The basis for the coding were the behavior change techniques identified by Michie et al. (2013) and the corresponding categorization (see Sect. 2.2.2), to which the specific mentions of the interviewees were assigned. To ensure the reliability of these assignments, the data were coded independently by two researchers and subsequently checked using intercoder agreement (Rädiker & Kuckartz, 2019).

4.3.2   Successful Measures from the Perspective of Those Affected

During the interviews, the affected individuals were asked to describe their experiences so far from the maintenance phase of lifestyle change. There was no specific inquiry into behavior change techniques identified as successful in the literature. This was to ensure that a broad, unbiased picture from the everyday life of the interviewees is presented.

The behavior change techniques identified through coding are given in brackets below. A detailed description can be found in Sect. 2.2.2.

In the area of nutrition, it was mentioned that specific guidelines and routines are helpful in adopting new eating habits. Interviewee 1 said: *"...I always cook the recipe after I have worked. I come home, cook, eat and then wait about three, four hours before I go to sleep"* (Behavioral goal, action planning, and habit formation). Those interviewees who used the Uplyfe program found the recipes particularly helpful as a useful guideline or as a concrete "roadmap" for healthy eating (Conserving mental resources). These and other respondents also expressed a desire for flexibility so as not to feel too restricted by the guidelines. Interviewee 2 expressed this as follows: *"And nothing is forbidden. I am allowed to eat dessert, when I am invited somewhere. Yes, then I just restrict myself again the next day."* Interviewee 3 also mentioned that he has developed a solid routine in terms of nutrition, but occasionally indulges himself. Interviewee 1 even deliberately planned a deviation from his newly developed healthy eating routine: *"I have set myself a goal that when I have lost 20 kilos, which I will soon, we will go for ice cream"* (Outcome goal and reward). These and similar statements suggest that a consistant framework is helpful for planning and maintaining a healthy diet, but at the same time it should not be too tight in order to sustain motivation.

Mindfulness when eating, i.e., a conscious focus on eating without parallel activities, was discussed by two respondents. Interviewee 5 puts it this way: *"When I eat alone, I can focus on the plate, what is on the plate and actually experience the food more consciously. Because the priority is eating"* (Remodeling the social environment). By eating more consciously, those affected better perceive when they are full and stop eating sooner.

A strategy for achieving and maintaining a sustainable healthy lifestyle, which was frequently mentioned in connection with both nutrition and exercise, is the formulation of goals. Stated goals primarily related to a behavior e.g., jogging three times a week (Behavioral goal), but sometimes also to an outcome, such as losing 20 kg in total within a defined time (Outcome goal). Especially with regard to outcome goals, several respondents expressed that the formulation of intermediate goals is helpful for them: *"I do have goals, but I take them step by step"* (Interview 2). Intermediate goals (graded tasks) and their review make deviations from planning apparent earlier (Self-monitoring), lead to motivation-enhancing successes more quickly, and in some respondents to a reward (Planning self-reward).

All respondents also reported routines in connection with exercise that they had created themselves (Building habits), e.g., by determining a fixed date at the gym or in their daily life: *"I have incorporated it, every hour I do my exercises"* (Interview 1). Three respondents also mentioned the beneficial effect of music, such as Interviewee 6: *"Exercise certainly helps and dancing makes you happy, music anyway"*. The group dynamics through exercise in a team or in group courses were also considered helpful (Unspecific social support). According to Interviewee 3, this is particularly due to words of praise from people in the group (Feedback on behavior).

Similar to the cooking recipes, a change was also desired in the exercise program. The respondents found an individual adaptation of the program particularly helpful, e.g., due to progress (Monitoring of results by external person) or based on health data such as lactate measurements (Biofeedback).

In terms of health, the respondents mainly mentioned improved well-being due to the successful lifestyle change, which motivated them to maintain the new behavior (Focus on previous successes). Interviewee 1 expressed this as follows: *"The awareness that I have made it and that it is therefore better to continue this way"*. Interviewee 5 also developed an improved body feeling through regular swimming and found this motivating. For Interviewee 3, it is mainly successes that motivate him to "stick with it". He visualizes this, for example, by comparing before and after photos and says that this gives him a "kick" (Self-monitoring of results and focus on previous successes). Equally important to him is "social support", which becomes clear in the following statement: *"I think something that is important—someone who supports you. Really getting you on track with small goals. Someone who maybe also supports you mentally"* (Emotional social support).

4.3.3   Frequently Used Behavior Change Techniques by Those Affected in the Maintenance Phase

The most frequently mentioned behavior change techniques were identified per interview, which are shown in Table 4.1. Since the survey aimed at successful behavior change techniques, this evaluation is based on the assumption that frequent mention indicates high relevance for sustainable success.

Across all interviews, the following behavior change techniques were mentioned most frequently in this order:

Table 4.1 Top 3 most frequently mentioned behavior change techniques per interview

	Interview 1	Interview 2	Interview 3	Interview 4	Interview 5	Interview 6	Interview 7
Top 1	Feedback	Regulation of negative emotions	Feedback	Social support	Goal setting	Social support	Behavior planning
Top 2	Behavior planning	Feedback	Reward	Feedback	Behavior practice	Behavior planning	Monitoring
Top 3	Goal setting	Goal setting	Social support	Behavior planning	Behavior planning	Regulation of negative emotions	Social support
	Reward		Behavior practice	Highlighting consequences			Feedback

1. Feedback,
2. Behavior planning,
3. Regulation of negative emotions,
4. Social support and
5. Goal setting.

It can be assumed that these are the techniques that, from the respondents' point of view, most successfully contribute to a sustainable lifestyle change.

A comparison of the results of sub-studies 1 and 2 shows a high level of consistency in the identified behavior change techniques. Goal setting, planning, and feedback are among the most successful behavior change techniques. Sub-study 1 also counted "practice of behavior" from the category "repetition and substitution" among the most successful behavior change techniques. Both techniques are also mentioned by the affected individuals (interviews 3 and 5), but they are not among the top 3 across all interviews. Compared to the experts, those affected consider social support to be more important.

4.4   Sub-study 3: Development of need-oriented Measures for a Sustainable Lifestyle Change

Answer to research question 3: How can the identified behavior change techniques be specifically designed as practical measures to support a sustainable lifestyle change?

4.4.1   Design Thinking Workshop with representatives of the health ecosystem

The final part of the study focused on the detailed specification and design of need-oriented measures for sustainable lifestyle changes, based on the identified behavior change techniques. For this purpose, a Design Thinking workshop was conducted with a total of six representatives from the health ecosystem. The participants included three employees of CSS, two employees of the family business Dr. Bähler Dropa, a network of over 100 pharmacies and drugstores, and an employee of the startup Uplyfe, which offers nutrition and exercise programs for a sustainable lifestyle change. All participants are employees of the three companies that accompanied this applied research project as business partners.

Using the approach of Human-centered Design based on IDEO (2018), the workshop aimed to develop solution ideas in the form of simple prototypes and then evaluate them. Human-centered design is understood as a design process that is divided into three phases: inspiration, ideation, and implementation. The *inspiration* phase focuses heavily on the needs of those people for whom a service is being designed. In the *ideation* phase, as many ideas as possible are then generated and presented in the form of very simple prototypes, tested, evaluated, and further developed. According to the Design Thinking approach by Tim Brown (2008), the goal of prototypes is to give new ideas a shape so that their strengths and weaknesses are easy to recognize and a basis for their further development is created. Prototypes should remain as reduced as possible to avoid unnecessary time or effort and thus keep the risks of misinvestments low. By reducing to the essentials, the central elements are put in the spotlight, so that feedback is received exactly on these elements. For services, for example, simple, short descriptions of scenarios can act as a prototype. These often represent a particularly valuable method for visualizing an idea because they put people at the center of the idea and listeners or viewers are less distracted by mechanical or aesthetic aspects when imagining the idea (Brown & Katz, 2019). In the *implementation* phase, the solution ideas are finally brought to market maturity.

4.4.2   Development of Prototype Need-Based Measures

The starting point of the inspiration phase in the present project were the interviews with those affected, described under Sect. 4.3. They served to understand the needs of those affected and to get an idea of their everyday life. In order for the workshop participants to develop empathy for those affected, a storytelling approach was chosen. Based on the interviews with those affected, three complementary personas were developed, from whose everyday life one of the researchers played out central sequences. These included a concrete design of the behavior change techniques identified as successful. From this, all participants worked out four idea sketches for measures or combinations of measures. This resulted in 24 very simple prototypes for health-promoting measures. The workshop participants briefly and succinctly presented their ideas to each other. They then evaluated these, with each person being able to distribute five points across all ideas, including their own. In human-centered design, the desirability of an idea, its feasibility, such as technical feasibility, and its viability are used as evaluation criteria. The participants evaluated these aspects based on their professional experience. This ensured that the prototypes were practice-relevant and implementable. This resulted in a pre-selection for further work with the prototypes at the end of the workshop.

The following selection of four practice-relevant, implementable measures answered the research question of how the identified behavior change techniques can be concretely designed as practical measures to support a sustainable lifestyle change:

1. Goal agreement: Customers agree on individual goals and are supported in achieving them through monthly checks
2. Rewards: Customers receive rewards, such as vouchers, after they have reached a defined target weight or made a behavior change, e.g., jogging once a week

3. Sponsor system: Customers have a supportive person in their environment who reminds them of their goals or with whom they can pursue goals together
4. Emergency button: Customers have the option at any time to report a relapse via a digital emergency button and receive support

The developed prototypes are only partially based on the behavior change techniques identified in sub-study 2, namely goal setting (goal setting) and regulation of negative emotions (emergency button). The mentor system is based on social support and thus on a behavior change technique that was identified in both previous sub-studies, but could not be counted among the most common behavior change techniques. The behavior change technique reward was only mentioned marginally in the previous sub-studies (affected interviews 1 and 3).

Following the workshop, the prototypes were further developed using a service concept detail sheet (Georgi et al., 2018) and the respective customer benefit was specified. This formed the basis for the development of the concrete app-based measures for the impact study described in chapter 5.

4.5 Conclusion

Across the three sub-studies presented, concrete measures for effectively supporting individuals in achieving sustainable lifestyle changes were identified, based on the most relevant techniques for those affected. These techniques include five of the 16 categories of behavior change techniques presented in Chap. 2 (Michie et al., 2013): "Goal setting and planning", "Feedback and monitoring", "Social support", "Regulation of negative emotions" and "Repetition and substitution". From this four practical measures were developed: goal setting, reward, sponsor system, and emergency button. The testing of these prototypes took place in the subsequent impact study described in Chap. 5.

References

Brown, T. (2008). Design thinking. *Harvard Business Review, 86*(6), 84.

Brown, T., & Katz, B. (2019). *Change by design: How design thinking transforms organizations and inspires innovation* (Revised and updated edition). Harper Business.

Deci, E. L., & Ryan, R. M. (2000). The "What" and "Why" of goal pursuits: Human needs and the self-determination of behavior. *Psychological Inquiry, 11*(4), 227–268. https://doi.org/10.1207/S15327965PLI1104_01.

Froschauer, U., & Lueger, M. (2020). *Das qualitative Interview: Zur Praxis interpretativer Analyse sozialer Systeme* (2. Aufl.). Facultas.

Georgi, D., Schäfer, A., Eichen, F., & Ahlers, M. (2018). Geschäftsmodellierung auf der Basis serviceorientierter Value Propositions – Toolbox. *Hochschule Luzern – Wirtschaft und Prof. Bruhn und Partner AG* (unveröffentlichtes Dokument).

IDEO. (2018). Facilitator's guide to introducing human centered design. https://www.designkit.org/resources/7.

Mayring, P. (2015). *Qualitative Inhaltsanalyse: Grundlagen und Techniken* (12. ed.). Beltz.

Michie, S., Richardson, M., Johnston, M., Abraham, C., Francis, J., Hardeman, W., Eccles, M. P., Cane, J., & Wood, C. E. (2013). The behavior change technique taxonomy (v1) of 93 hierarchically clustered techniques: Building an international consensus for the reporting of behavior change interventions. *Annals of Behavioral Medicine, 46*(1), 81–95. https://doi.org/10.1007/s12160-013-9486-6.

Przyborski, A., & Wohlrab-Sahr, M. (2021). *Qualitative Sozialforschung: Ein Arbeitsbuch* (5. Aufl.). De Gruyter.

Rädiker, S., & Kuckartz, U. (Eds.). (2019). Intercoder-Übereinstimmung analysieren. *Analyse qualitativer Daten mit MAXQDA* (S. 287–303). Springer. https://doi.org/10.1007/978-3-658-22095-2_19.

The Diabetes Prevention Program Research Group. (2002). The DIABETES PREVENTION PROGRAM (DPP): Description of lifestyle intervention. *Diabetes Care, 25*(12), 2165–2171. https://doi.org/10.2337/diacare.25.12.2165.

Acceptance of Motivation-Oriented Behavior Change Techniques and Relevance of the Actors in the Ecosystem

Contents

A. Schäfer et al., *Maintaining a Healthy Lifestyle*,
https://doi.org/10.1007/978-3-662-69460-2_5

Abstract

This chapter summarizes the basics, methodology, and results of a study on the acceptance of different digital behavior change techniques and the relevance of various actors in the health care ecosystem. The starting point is the assumption that only accepted measures contribute to sustainable behavior change. The results show that measures based on the behavior change technique of goal setting and monitoring enjoy relatively high acceptance. The measure that is oriented towards autonomous motivation is always preferred. The study provides indications of factors that influence the acceptance of the different behavior change techniques. With regard to the actors in the ecosystem, a clear picture emerges: Doctors, family members, and/or people in the same household have the greatest relevance in maintaining a healthy lifestyle.

The increasing digitization is also of high relevance in the health sector. Therefore, the present study examines the effectiveness of digital behavior change techniques. The starting point of the empirical study is the assumption that a sustainablebehavior change can only be supported by measures that are also accepted by those affected, i.e., perceived as useful and used.

First, an explanation of the relevant basics for the effectiveness and acceptance of digital measures to support a sustainable lifestyle change in the health sector is given. This includes describing which digital behavior change techniques have proven effective in clinical studies. Based on this, the research questions of the empirical study in connection with the use and acceptance of digital measures are developed and explained. Furthermore, the basics of the relevance of different actors in the ecosystem are discussed and a corresponding research question is derived. This is followed by an explanation of the procedures and finally, the results are summarized.

5.1   Basics and Research Questions

5.1.1   Effectiveness of Digital Measures

Digital measures contribute to promoting healthy behavior and have various advantages over traditional face-to-face measures. Digital measures are cost-effective and can be used flexibly and time-savingly, as, for example, scheduling and travel time to health specialists are eliminated (Arigo et al., 2019). This makes it easier to apply a measure continuously and maintain healthy behaviors sustainably. In lifestyle changes towards more exercise and healthier nutrition, it is particularly important that the measures are maintained over a longer period of time, as weight loss often results in a yo-yo effect and thus a renewed weight gain (Sharpe et al., 2017). In order for a digital measure to effectively and sustainably support those affected in their health-promoting behavior, it is necessary to empirically investigate its effectiveness (van Vugt et al., 2013).

Measures for a change towards a healthy lifestyle with more exercise and healthy nutrition are diverse and can consist of a variety of different approaches. The 16 different categories of behavior change techniques (BCTs) developed by Michie et al. (2013) summarize all techniques that lead to a behavior change (see Chap. 2). A behavior change technique is defined as the smallest active component of an intervention, i.e., a set of activities aimed at changing behavior. Behavior change techniques can be applied alone or in combination.

Studies show that measures that include behavior change techniques are generally effective in behavior changes in the health sector (Carraça et al., 2021; Samdal et al., 2017; van Vugt et al., 2013). A meta-analysis examined the effectiveness of behavior change techniques in promoting a healthy lifestyle, i.e., more exercise and healthy nutrition, in overweight adults (Samdal et al., 2017). A distinction was made between short-term and long-term behavior changes. The number of behavior change techniques had a positive influence on long-term behavior changes: the more that were integrated, the more effective the measures were. In addition, the following specific behavior change techniques proved effective in long-term behavior changes:

- Behavioral goal (Category 1: Goal setting and planning)
- Outcome goal (Category 1: Goal setting and planning)
- Self-monitoring of behavior (Category 2: Feedback and monitoring)
- Feedback on outcomes (Category 2: Feedback and monitoring)
- Graded tasks (Category 8: Reppetition and substation)
- Adding helpful objects to the environment (Category 12: Antecedents)

In another meta-analysis, the effectiveness of behavior change techniques in digital and analog measures to promote exercise in overweight adults was examined (Carraça et al., 2021). A total of 62 studies were considered that included measures with at least one behavior change technique and examined the effectiveness of 56 behavior change techniques. The effectiveness differed between digital measures and measures that were conveyed face-to-face. In the case of digital measures, the following four behavior change techniques had a positive influence on the promotion of exercise:

- Behavioral goal (Category 1: Goal setting and planning)
- Outcome goal (Category 1: Goal setting and planning)
- Graded tasks (Category 8: Repeat and substitute)
- Social reward for behavior (Category 10: Reward)

The behavior change technique *Self-Monitoring of Behaviors* (Category 2: Feedback and Monitoring) had a negative effect on promoting physical activity. In another meta-analysis, inconsistent effects for self-monitoring were found across various studies (Hennessy

et al., 2020). These different findings can be explained by the fact that the health parameters examined in the studies vary (e.g., weight loss or promotion of physical activity)
and different target groups were included in the study (e.g., overweight adults or general adult population). Another meta-analysis examined the effect of behavior change
techniques used in web-based measures in people with diabetes (van Vugt et al., 2013).
The effect of behavior change techniques on different health parameters was considered:
effect on health-relevant behavior (e.g., exercise or nutrition), on clinical parameters
(e.g., blood sugar or cholesterol) and on psychological factors (e.g., self-efficacy or well-
being). In the 13 studies analyzed, a total of 33 behavior change techniques were identified. The rather small number of included studies may be due to the fact that at the time
of the meta-analysis, digitally based measures were not yet widely used. A large number
of the behavior change techniques examined had a positive effect on health:

- Feedback on results (Category 2: Feedback and Monitoring)
- Information about health consequences (Category 5: Consequences of Behavior)
- Problem solving (Category 1: Goal Setting and Planning)
- Self-monitoring of behavior (Category 2: Feedback and Monitoring)
- Self-monitoring of results (Category 2: Feedback and Monitoring)

Digital measures based on behavior change techniques can thus support individuals with
health problems in making behavior changes towards a healthy lifestyle.

5.1.2 Influence of the Design of Measures on Acceptance

For a digital measure to be effective, it must be accepted and used by the target groups.
Sharpe et al. (2017) examined in a review of qualitative and quantitative studies which
factors from the users' perspective promote interaction with digital measures for weight
reduction. Different types of digital tools were examined: web-based tools, apps, and
SMS reminders. The study differentiated between factors that influence the download or
initial use of a tool and factors that influence continuous use. The following discussion
will only cover the latter factors:

- *Customizability:* The customizability of a measure, such as individual feedback and
  individually tailored information, has a positive effect on its use. Customization
  allows the measure to be better integrated into everyday life. A non-customizable
  measure, on the other hand, can appear impersonal and generic.
- *Social Support:* The possibility for social interactions within a digital program
  shows mixed effects. On the one hand, social support is desired because it allows for
  exchange with people who are in a similar situation. Online forums can create a sense
  of community. In addition, social comparisons can be motivating. On the other hand,
  online forums are the least popular features of a digital program, as they can appear

unreliable if the desired support is not provided. Popularity is therefore dependent on the activity on the online platforms.

- *Feedback and Motivation:* Regular feedback is appreciated by users and perceived as motivating. Regular encouragements also support effective behavior changes. However, it must be ensured that such digital features do not appear impersonal or too repetitive.
- *Ease of Installation and Use:* If a digital measure is easy to set up and use, this promotes continuous use.
- *Self-Monitoring and Reminders:* Featuress that allow users to observe their own behavior and progress are important for users. Regular reminders and notifications also prove to be relevant for effective behavior changes.
- *Knowledge Transfer:* Easy access to relevant content is important for the users and an added value of digital solutions. Thus, knowledge transfer and practical tips can support effective behavior change.

A user-friendly design of the digital measure, tailored to the needs of the users, is essential for it to be accepted and used by potential users.

Against the background outlined, the following questions arise for the present research project: *Which digital measures lead to higher acceptance among target groups? (Research question 1) What are the influencing factors on the intention to use measures? (Research question 2).*

5.1.3   Significance of Autonomous Motivation for the Maintenance of Behavioral Changes

Various studies have dealt with the correlations between motivation and behavioral change (e.g., Ryan et al., 2021). These show that behavioral changes in the health context are more successful when they occur due to autonomous motivation (Ng et al., 2012). If healthy behavior is to be maintained in the long term, it is important that it does not arise from controlled motivation—i.e., motivation from outside—but from autonomous motivation (Ryan et al., 2007). With autonomous motives, an action is perceived as voluntary and carried out on one's own initiative, e.g., out of joy in the action. With controlled motives, an action is perceived as imposed from outside and carried out due to an external drive, e.g., due to a reward (Hagger et al., 2020).

Therefore, the present study aims to investigate to what extent the design of the measures in an autonomous and controlled form influences acceptance and thus also the willingness to use. On this basis, the following research question is formulated for the present study: *Do autonomy oriented digital measures lead to higher acceptance among th e target group? (Research question 3).*

5.1.4 Insights into the Relevance of Actors in the Ecosystem

In relation to the relevance of actors in the ecosystem, different dimensions of relevance are distinguished. The present study focuses on the dimension of conveying relevant information and the support tailored to those affected. A distinction of these two dimensions allows a differentiated view regarding the justification of relevance. Access to information can be a basis for better-informed decisions and thus have a positive effect on relationships with the various actors within the ecosystem (Beirão et al., 2017). At the same time, it can be assumed that individual actors within the ecosystem are relevant to those affected because they offer support tailored to the needs of those potential users. Accordingly, actors can be differentiated as to whether they are more relevant in terms of information transmission and/or tailored support.

The study aims to answer the following research question: *Which actors in the ecosystem are relevant from the perspective of the target groupsfor maintaining a healthy lifestyle? (Research question 4).*

5.2 Procedures and Methods of the Survey

In a survey, nearly 400 people who wanted to change or maintain their lifestyle for health reasons evaluated different digital measures for lifestyle change. The goal was to assess the acceptance and the intention to use of differently designed measures.

5.2.1 Participants with a Desire for Lifestyle Change for Health Reasons

For the survey, individuals from the German-speaking part of Switzerland were recruited via a market research panel. Only individuals who wanted to achieve or maintain a healthy lifestyle for health reasons, e.g., overweight, high blood pressure, or diabetes, were considered. A healthy lifestyle was defined as a lifestyle with sufficient exercise and healthy nutrition. Due to these strict selection criteria, 354 individuals had to be excluded from the survey. In total, 411 individuals completed the survey completely. 14 individuals were excluded from the evaluation because they showed an inconsistent response pattern, indicating that they may not have filled out the survey seriously. The final sample included the evaluation of a total of 397 individuals.

The participants were between 25 and 82 years old. The average age was 62 years. Compared to the average age in the Swiss population of 42 years (Federal Statistical Office, 2020), the sample was significantly older. This is due to the fact that the health problems examined occur more frequently with increasing age. With 199 women and 198 men, a balanced gender distribution of the sample was achieved.

Table 5.1 Examined measures to promote a healthy lifestyle

Motivation orientation		
Autonomous	**Controlled**	**None**
1a) Goal setting: Set goals yourself	1b) Goal setting: Health coach sets goals	—
2a) Monitoring: Own daily goal	2b) Monitoring: Compare daily goal with others	—
3a) Challenge: Own weekly challenge	3b) Challenge: Joint challenge with others	—
4a) Social support: Personal buddy	4b) Social support: Community	—
—	—	5) Share progress
—	—	6) Emergency button

5.2.2 Digital Measures with Autonomous and Controlled Motivation Orientation

The participants evaluated ten measures to promote a healthy lifestyle (see Table 5.1). The measures are based on six behavior change techniques. The selection of the underlying behavior change techniques was based on studies on the effectiveness of digital measures. Only behavior change techniques were selected that have proven effective in achieving health goals in the studies. Furthermore, a subset of six behavior change techniques was selected and tested based on the workshop with experts (see Chap. 4).

The concrete design of the measures was also based on the workshop with experts explained in Sect. 4.4. Four behavior change techniques were implemented into two concrete measures with different motivation orientations—autonomous and controlled. In the case of autonomous motivation orientation, the specific design of the measure is determined by the users themselves. Since they are responsible for the specific design of the measures and have to motivate themselves for the implementation, this requires a stronger expression of autonomous motives. In the case of controlled motivation orientation, the measures are oriented towards support from external parties. These are experts such as a personal health coach who suggests personalized measures, or also people from the personal social environment. By integrating external people, these measures address controlled motives more strongly. The measures were visualized and presented in the style of an app. Each measure represents a digital featureof a fictitious app.

Goal Setting
In the measure Goal Agreement, goals are defined regarding healthy nutrition and exercise (see Fig. 5.1). The goal setting corresponds to the behavior change technique *1.1 Behavioral Goal* Setting (Michie et al., 2013): A goal is set that describes a behavior. In the autonomous version, these are set by the users themselves; in the controlled version, the goals are set by a personal health coach.

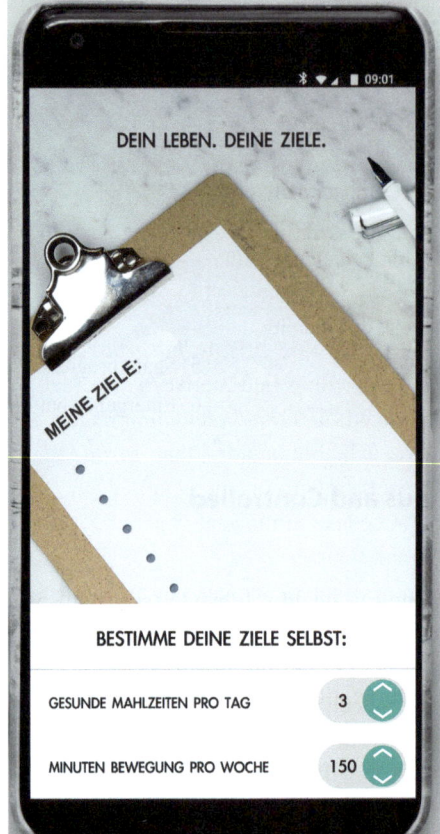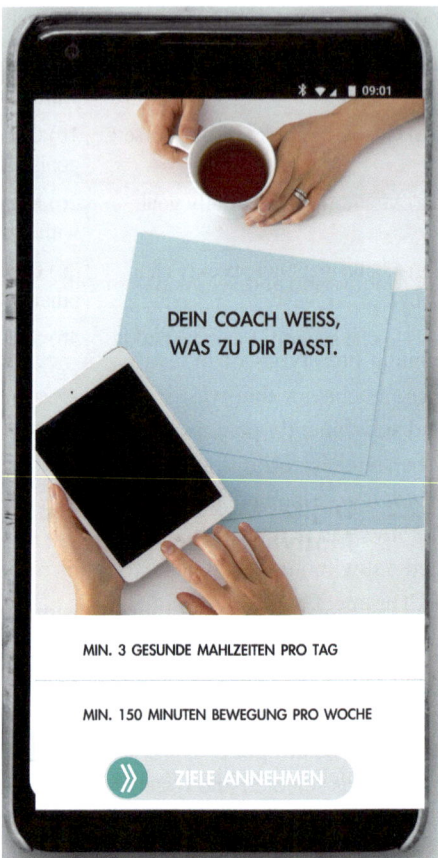

Fig. 5.1 Measure Goal Setting: autonomous version = left; controlled version = right. (Images courtesy of: Markus Winkler, Unsplash; Avel Chuklanov, Unsplash)

Monitoring

The measure Monitoring provides information about a set goal (see Fig. 5.2). This measure is based on the behavior change technique *2.3 Self-Monitoring of Behavior* (Michie et al., 2013): The behavior is recorded by the person concerned. In the autonomous version, the individuals compare their progress in relation to the goals they have set themselves. In the controlled version, one compares oneself in relation to other participants within the health app.

Challenge

In the measure Challenge, a weekly challenge is defined (see Fig. 5.3). The Challenge corresponds to the behavior change technique *1.4 Action Planning* (Michie et al., 2013): The execution of a behavior is planned in detail. In the autonomous version, this corresponds to a challenge that is carried out alone. In the controlled version, the challenge is carried out together with another person.

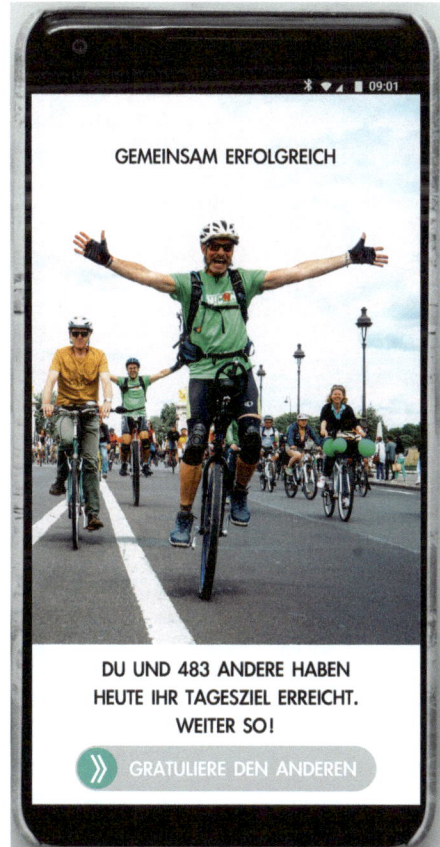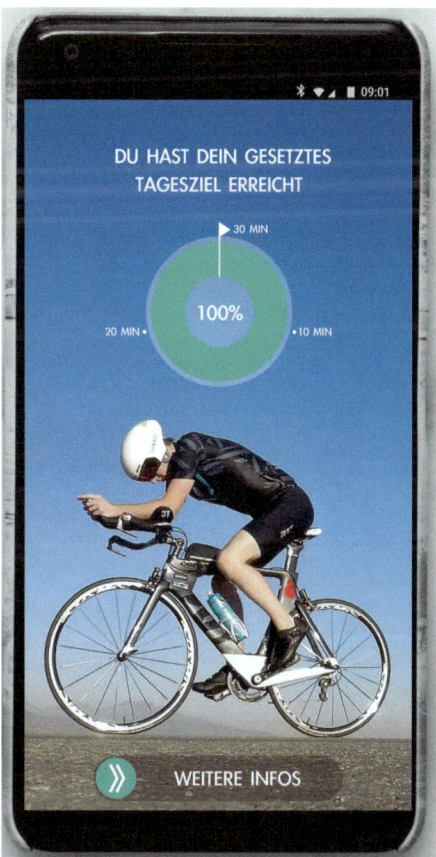

Fig. 5.2 Measure Monitoring: autonomous version = left; controlled version = right. (Images courtesy of: Beau Runsten, Unsplash; Fred Pixlab, Unsplash)

Social Support

In the measure Social Support, a person is designated who supports one in achieving the goals (see Fig. 5.4). This measure corresponds to the behavior change technique *3.2 Practical Social Support* (Michie et al., 2013): The person concerned receives practical support from a reference person. In the autonomous version, one chooses a so-called buddy from one's own social environment. In the controlled version, one receives support from the community of the health app.

Sharing Progress

In the Measure Share Progress, the progress in achieving personal goals can be shared on social media. This measure corresponds to the behavior change technique *6.2 Social Comparison* (Michie et al., 2013): A comparison with other people is encouraged

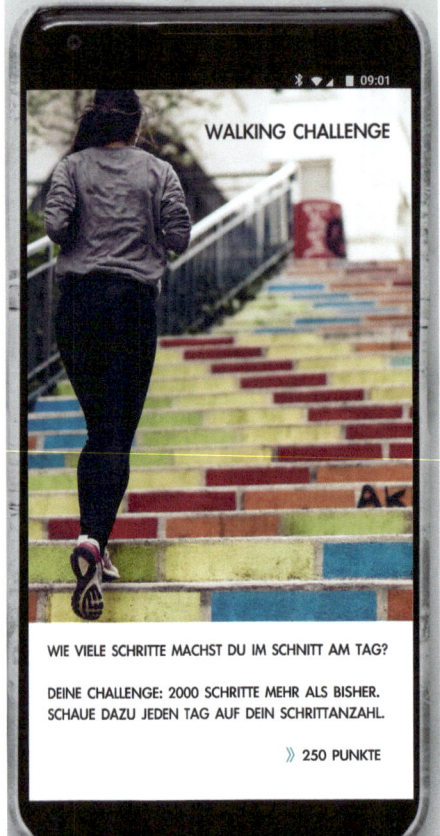 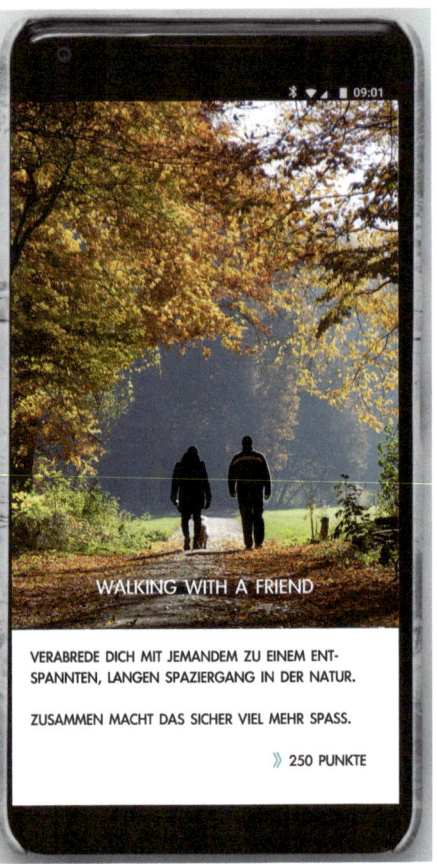

Fig. 5.3 Measure Challenge: autonomous version = left; controlled version = right. (Images courtesy of: Ev, Unsplash; Shaojie, Unsplash)

to compare one's own performance with others. This measure does not differentiate between autonomous and controlled motivation orientation (see Fig. 5.5).

Emergency Button

The Measure Emergency Button is designed to provide support when encountering challenges or obstacles in achieving personal health goals. This measure corresponds to the behavior change technique *3.1 Social Support (unspecific)* (Michie et al., 2013): The user receives social support without specific details about the form of support. This measure also does not differentiate between autonomous and controlled motivation orientation (see Fig. 5.6).

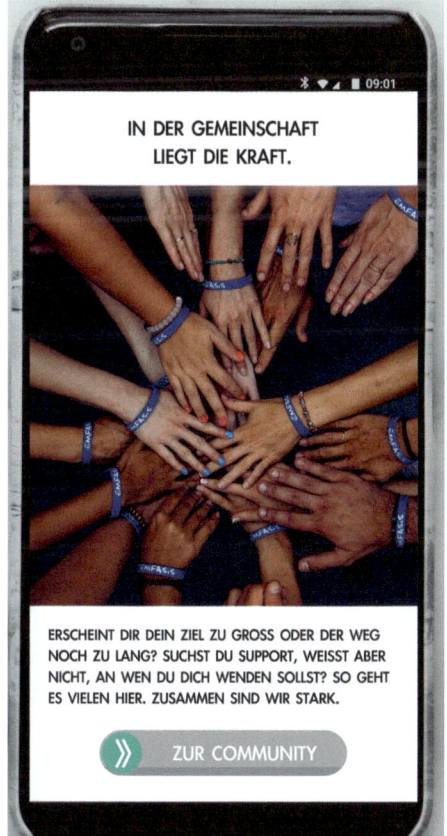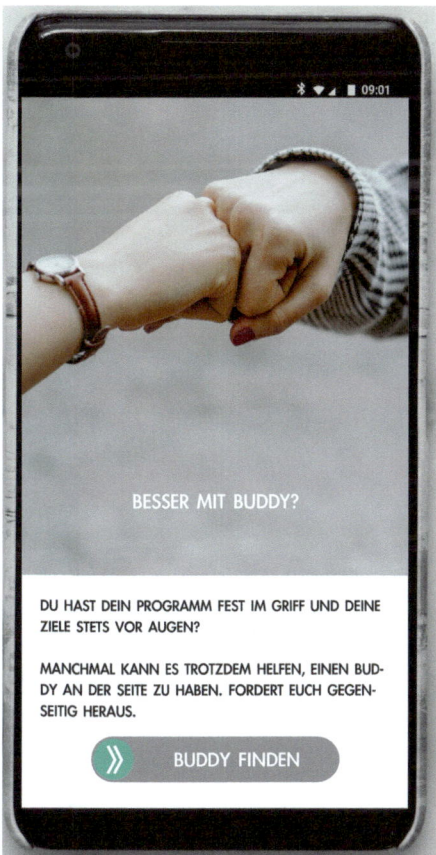

Fig. 5.4 Measure Social Support: autonomous version = left; controlled version = right. (Images courtesy of: Ashkan Forouzani, Unsplash; Perry Grone, Unsplash)

5.2.3   Assessment of Acceptance and Intention to Use Digital Measures

The participants evaluated the measures based on several characteristics, which represent various facets of acceptance, and their intention to use. The following characteristics were used to assess acceptance: *Fun* ("I would enjoy using this fnature[1]."), *Ease of Use* ("The feature would be easy for me to use"), *Usefulness* ("This feature would be useful for me") and *Suitability for everyday use* ("The feature could be easily integrated into

---

[1] In the survey, the term digital feature was always used for the individual digital measures. At the beginning of the survey, it was explained that a fictitious health app is being examined, which has different digital features.

Fig. 5.5 Measure Share Progress. (Image courtesy of: Jenny Hill, Unsplash)

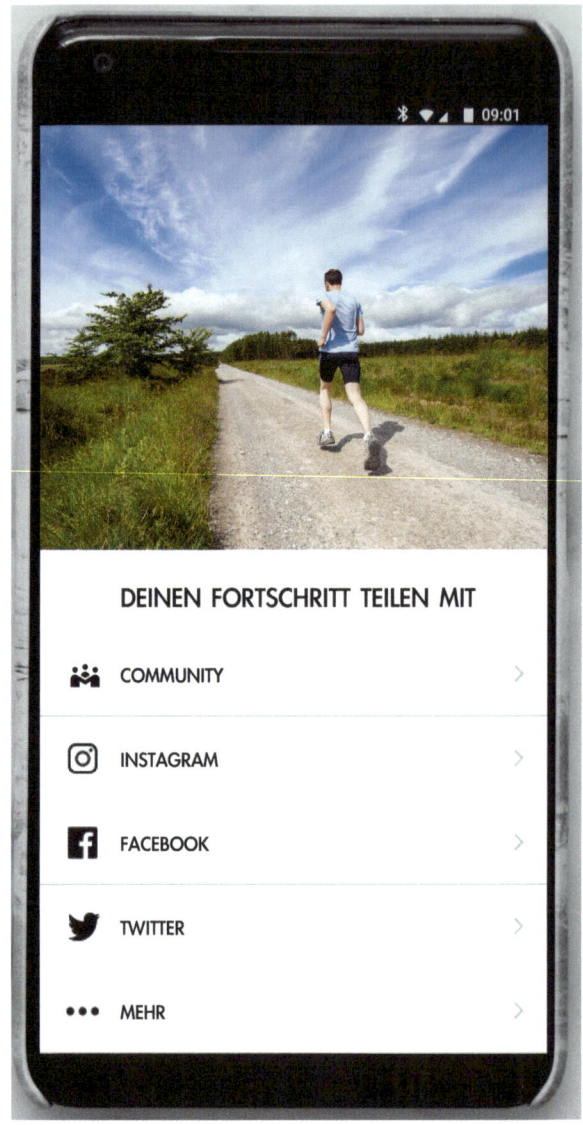

my daily routine"). The intention to use was assessed with one item ("I would use this feature"). After evaluating all measures, the general interest in a health app with such features was measured ("All things considered: How high is your interest in using such a health app with various features, such as setting goals […], as part of a health program?"). The participants indicated their agreement with the statements on a 7-point scale from 1 ("Strongly disagree") to 7 ("Strongly agree").

Fig. 5.6 Measure Emergency
Button. (Image courtesy of:
Lidia Estaban, Unsplash)

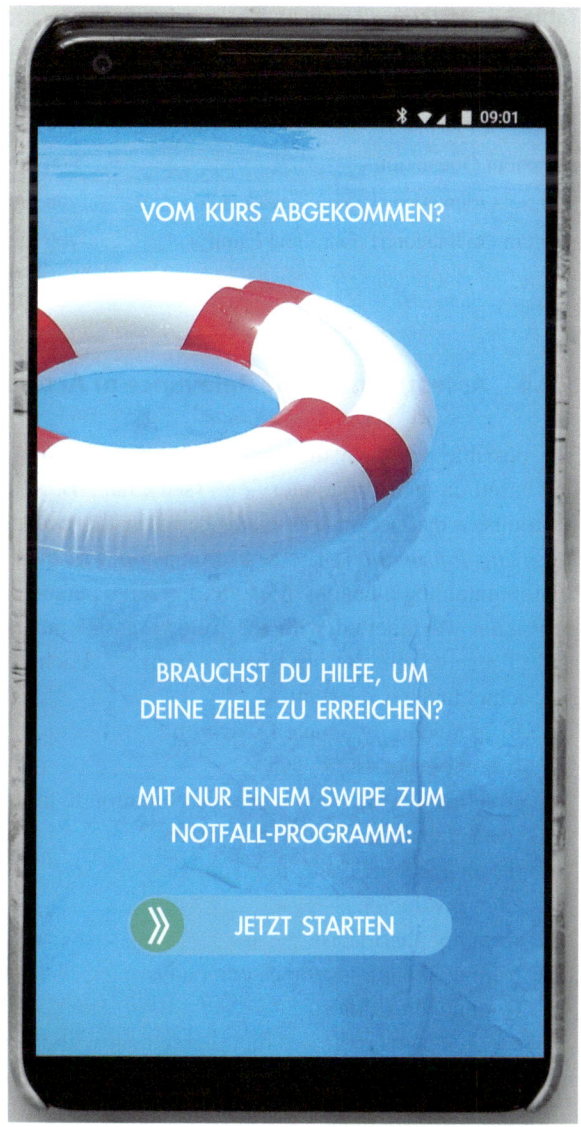

The participants' motivation orientation was assessed using a specially adapted short version of the Health Causality Orientations Scale (Smit & Bol, 2020). The HCOS is based on the General Causality Orientations Scale by Deci and Ryan (1985), which was adapted to the health context. It assesses to what extent a person's motivation to change their health behavior is intrinsic or extrinsic (motivated through professionals or through friends and family). In the present survey, the motivation orientation was assessed with one question each (see Table 5.2).

Table 5.2 Motivation Orientation (adapted short version according to Smit & Bol, 2020)

Motivation Orientation	Item
In the past, when you had to motivate yourself to do something for your health, how likely would you say it was that…	
Autonom Orientation	… you found the motivation yourself?
Control Orientation (Professionals)	… you turned to an expert to motivate you?
Control Orientation (Friends and Family)	… you turned to friends and family to motivate you?

5.2.4   Assessment of the Relevance of Actors in the Ecosystem

The possible actors in the ecosystem for maintaining a healthy lifestyle were identi-fied based on qualitative interviews (see Chap. 4). Since the actors can take on different functions, a distinction was made between the two dimensions *Receiving Support* and *Receiving Information*. The first dimension was queried with the following statement: "For maintaining a healthy lifestyle, I receive personalized support from…". The second dimension was queried with the following statement: "For maintaining a healthy life-style, I receive relevant information from…". Each statement was followed by a list of nine actors in the ecosystem:

…from my family/people I live with.
…from my friends.
…from people who are in a similar situation to me.
…from clubs/fitness studios or similar.
…through technical aids (e.g., apps).
…from my doctor.
…from my pharmacist.
…from my health insurance company.
…from my nutritionist.

The participants indicated their agreement with the respective statements on a 7-point scale from 1 ("Strongly disagree") to 7 ("Strongly agree").

5.3   Results

5.3.1   Intended Use of Digital Measures for Lifestyle Change

In Fig. 5.7, the measures are arranged in descending order of intended use. The respond-ents would most likely use monitoring with their own daily goal (autonomous motivation orientation), goal setting where goals can be set by themselves (autonomous motivation

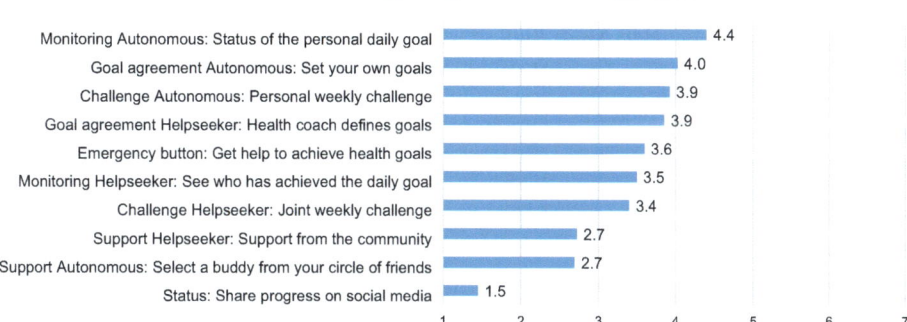

Agreement with the statement «I would use this function.» (n = 397). » Mean values on a
Scale from 1= «Strongly disagree» to 7= «Strongly agree».

Fig. 5.7 Intended Use of Digital Measures for Lifestyle Change

orientation), and the challenge that is carried out alone (autonomous motivation orientation). Therefore, in the overall comparison, measures from the categories of goal setting and monitoring show the greatest willingness to use and thus the highest acceptance. Acceptance is lower for measures with social comparison and social support.

In general, the participants indicate that they would rather use measures with autonomous motivation orientation than measures with controlled motivation orientation. Overall the affected persons would make little use of measures for social support and the opportunity to share their own progress.

5.3.2   Intention to use Digital Measures with Autonomous and Controlled Motivation Orientation

It was investigated whether there are differences in the intention to use between measures with autonomous motivation orientation and measures with controlled motivation orientation. For this purpose, the two measures with different motivation orientations were compared using a t-test. Table 5.3 shows the results of these comparisons. A reading example: The measure goal setting with autonomous motivation orientation (setting goals oneself) has an average intention to use of 4.02 on a scale of 1 to 7. The measure goal setting with controlled motivation orientation (health coach sets goals) has an average intention to use of 3.85. This difference is statistically significant at a level of $p < .05$. Overall, the result show that all measures with autonomous motivation orientation would be used more by the respondents than those with a controlled motivation orientation.

Table 5.3 Comparison of the intention to use measures with autonomous and controlled motivation orientation (N = 397)

Measure	Autonomous Motivation Orientation		Controlled Motivation Orientation	
	Average	Standard Deviation	Average	Standard Deviation
Goal Setting	4.02	1.84	3.85*	1.81
Monitoring	4.39	1.83	3.49**	1.89
Challenge	3.92	1.88	3.39**	1.87
Social Support	2.69	1.68	2.72	1.73

Note. * = statistically significant at level p <. 05, ** = statistically significant at level p <.0 1. Scale: 1 = Strongly disagree; 7 = Strongly agree

5.3.3   Factors Influencing the Intention to use Digital Measures with Motivation-oriented Design

Using regression analysis, it was investigated to what extent the assessment of the properties of digital measures is related to the intention to use. The results of the regression analyses of the measures with motivation-oriented design are presented below. Positive correlations mean: The more the measure is perceived as fun, easy, useful, or suitable for everyday use, the more likely the measure would be used. Negative correlations mean: The more the measure is perceived as fun, easy, useful, or suitable for everyday use, the less likely the measure would be used.

Goal Setting
Regarding the measure of goal setting, the fun shows the greatest statistically significant correlation with the intention to use, regardless of whether the measure is designed autonomy oriented or controlled (see Table 5.4). Perceived usefulness and everyday applicability also show a significant correlation with the intention to use both measures, with everyday applicability showing a greater correlation for the controlled goal setting

Table 5.4 Factors influencing the intention to use the goal setting measure

Influencing Factor	Autonomous Goal Setting: Beta Coefficient	Controlled Goal Setting: Beta Coefficient
(Intercept)	(−0.411)	(−0.447)
Fun	0.534**	0.624**
Ease of use	0.008	0.007
Usefulness	0.256**	0.129**
Suitability for everyday use	0.227**	0.304**

Note. * = statistically significant at level p <. 05, ** = statistically significant at level p < .01

Table 5.5 Factors influencing the intention to use the monitoring measure

Influencing factor	Autonomous monitoring: Beta coefficient	Controlled monitoring: Beta coefficient
(Intercept)	(–0.323)	(–0.328)
Fun	0.567**	0.644**
Ease of use	–0.128**	–0.074*
Usefulness	0.210**	0.226**
Suitability for everyday use	0.374**	0.221**

Note. *=statistically significant at level p <. 05, **=statistically significant at level p < .01

Table 5.6 Influencing factors on the intention to use the measure Challenge

Influencing factor	Autonomous Challenge: Beta Coefficient	Controlled Challenge: Beta Coefficient
(Intercept)	(–0.257)	(–0.316)
Fun	0.515**	0.539**
Ease of use	–0.107*	–0.016
Usefulness	0.210**	0.320**
Suitability for everyday use	0.391**	0.164**

Note. *=statistically significant at level p <.05, **=statistically significant at level p <.01

compared to the autonomy oriented goal setting. In both measures, the ease of use does not show a significant correlation with the intention to use.

Monitoring
All four properties have a statistically significant relationship with the intention to use the monitoring measure, regardless of their motivation orientation (see Table 5.5). For both measures, the fun has the greatest relationship with the intention to use. In autonomy oriented monitoring, suitability for everyday use shows a rather large relationship with the intention to use, while usefulness shows a medium relationship. In controlled monitoring, both usefulness and suitability to everyday use have a medium relationship. Ease of Use shows a small negative relationship with the intention to use, i.e., the more the measure is perceived as easy to use, the *lower* is the intention to use.

Challenge
In the autonomy oriented challenge, a statistically significant correlation with the intention to use was demonstrated for all four properties. However, in the controlled challenge, the factor ease of use is not significant (see Table 5.6). In both challenges, the fun shows the greatest correlation with the intention to use. In the autonomous challenge, the

Table 5.7 Factors influencing the intention to use the measure of social support

Influencing factor	Social support autonomous: Beta coefficient	Social support controlled: Beta coefficient
(Intercept)	(–0.052)	(–0.107)
Fun	0.576**	0.560**
Ease of use	–0.029	–0.103**
Usefulness	0.266**	0.292**
Everyday applicability	0.105*	0.216**

Note. * = statistically significant at level p <.05, ** = statistically significant at level p <.01

suitability for everyday use also has a large correlation with the intention to use, whereas in the controlled challenge, the usefulness shows a rather large correlation with the intention to use. Ease of use is characterized by only a small negative correlation to usage intention in the autonomous challenge, i.e., the more the measure is perceived as easy to use, the *lower* is the intention to use.

Social Support

In the case of controlled social support, all four characteristics show a statistically significant correlation, while in the case of autonomy oriented social support, the factor ease of use is not significant (see Table 5.7). In both measures, fun has the greatest correlation with the intention to use. In addition, usefulness and suitability for everyday use show a medium correlation with the intention to use. In the case of controlled social support, there is also a negative correlation between ease of use and the intention to use, i.e., the more the measure is perceived as easy to use, the *lower* is the intention to use.

5.3.4   Relevance of the Actors in the Ecosystem from the Perspective of the Target Groups

Overall, there are no significant differences between the two dimensions of receiving support (see Fig. 5.8) and receiving information (see Fig. 5.9) from actors in the ecosystem. The ranking of relevance is identical for both dimensions: Medical professionals have the highest average relevance when it comes to maintaining a healthy lifestyle, closely followed by people living in the same household. With an agreement between 4.3 and 5.2 on a scale of 1 to 7, the cooperation with these actors is positively evaluated. The least relevance is given to fitness studios and nutritionists.

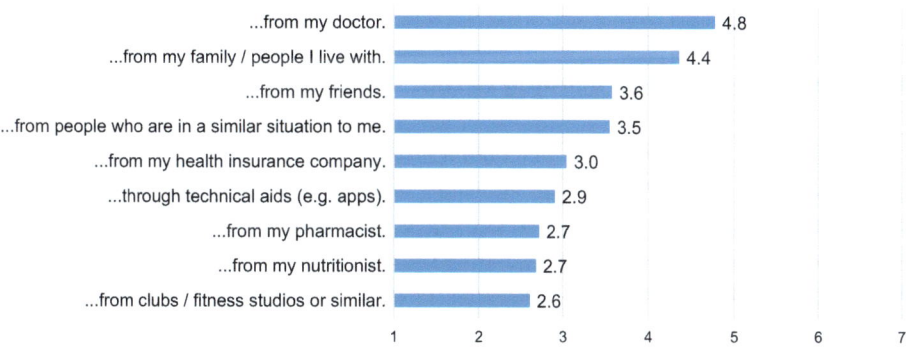

Fig. 5.8 Relevance of the actors in the ecosystem: Receiving support. Average values on a scale of 1 to 7

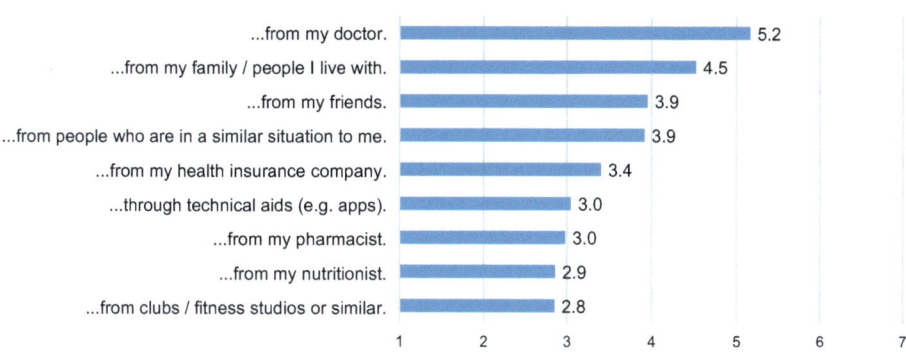

Fig. 5.9 Relevance of the actors in the ecosystem: Receiving information. Average values on a scale of 1 to 7

5.4   Conclusion and Answering of the Research Questions

The conclusion is structured along the four research questions of the study.

5.4.1   Digital Measures Leading to Higher Acceptance

To answer research question 1 *(Which digital measures lead to higher acceptance?)*, the following can be stated. Overall, the measures of goal setting and monitoring have the highest acceptance. This suggests that corresponding digital offers successfully support those affected in maintaining a healthy lifestyle. It is surprising that goal setting measures also has a relatively high acceptance in maintaining a new lifestyle, as goal setting often stands at the beginning of a behavior change. Social support is not very popular. Also, the potential users would very rarely use the opportunity to share successes in the group.

5.4.2   Acceptance of Autonomy Oriented Digital Measures

Research question 2 *(Do autonomy oriented digital measures lead to higher acceptance?)* can be summarized as follows. The measures of goal setting, monitoring, and challenge have a significantly higher intention to use in the case of autonomous motivational orientation than in the case of controlled motivational orientation. Only in the case of the measure of social support is there no difference between the two versions. This measure differs from the others in that support from external persons per se is associated with less autonomy.

Digital measures would be used primarily when they promote the users' autonomy. When designing digital measures, care should be taken to develop digital features that can be used independently and without the involvement of third parties. In this way, those affected can be supported in their autonomy on the way to a healthy lifestyle with digital measures.

5.4.3   Factors Influencing Willingness to Use and Acceptance

Regarding the question of the factors influencing the willingness to use and acceptance (research question 3), the study demonstrates that for all measures, regardless of the motivational orientation, the factor fun has the greatest correlation with the intention to use. For three measures (goal setting controlled, monitoring autonomous, challenge autonomous), a large correlation with the intention to use could also be demonstrated for everyday suitability. For the measure Social Support with controlled motivational orientation, the usefulness also has a rather large correlation with the intention to use.

For ease of use, a negative correlation with the intention to use can be found for four measures (monitoring autonomous, monitoring controlled, challenge autonomous, social support controlled), i.e., the simpler the measure is perceived to be in use, the *less* it would actually be used. However, the correlations are rather small. There are no systematic differences between measures with autonomous and controlled motivational orientation.

For digital measures to be accepted by users, the use of a digital feature should primarily be fun. It is also important that the digital feature can be well integrated into everyday life. The ease of use of a measure is less relevant and may even have a negative impact on acceptance and use. This could be explained by the fact that a digital measure should also be exciting maybe through more complexity.

In general, it can be stated that the emotional factor plays a central role in the concrete design of a digital measure for health promotion and should therefore be taken into account. This is in line with the findings from the literature on gamification, which attribute a central importance to the emotional factor in the context of digital support for lifestyle changes (DeSmet et al., 2014; Graesser et al., 2009).

5.4.4 Relevant Actors in the Ecosystem for Maintaining a Healthy Lifestyle

Finally, in answer to research question 4 *(Which actors in the ecosystem are relevant from the perspective of the target groups for maintaining a healthy lifestyle?)*, it can be stated that the greatest relevance in maintaining a healthy lifestyle lies with doctors. Almost equally relevant are family members and/or people in the same household. With regard to the design of the ecosystem, the present study confirms that even in the maintenance stage, traditionally trained medical professionals play a major role. The further development of an ecosystem that takes into account the importance of these stakeholders can contribute to value creation.

In addition, the relevance of important actors such as pharmacies or nutritionists, as indicated by the participants, clearly lags behind their potential. For the further development of the health ecosystem with the goal of maintaining a healthy lifestyle, it is recommended to raise the awareness and relevance of these actors and to integrate them into the health care ecosystem.

References

Arigo, D., Jake-Schoffman, D. E., Wolin, K., Beckjord, E., Hekler, E. B., & Pagoto, S. L. (2019). The history and future of digital health in the field of behavioral medicine. *Journal of Behavioral Medicine, 42*(1), 67–83. https://doi.org/10.1007/s10865-018-9966-z.

Beirão, G., Patrício, L., & Fisk, R. P. (2017). Value cocreation in service ecosystems: Investigating health care at the micro, meso, and macro levels. *Journal of Service Management, 28*(2), 227–249. https://doi.org/10.1108/JOSM-11-2015-0357.

Bundesamt für Statistik. (2020). Durchschnittsalter der ständigen Wohnbevölkerung nach Staatsangehörigkeitskategorie, Geschlecht und Kanton, 2010–2020. https://www.bfs.admin.ch/bfs/de/home/statistiken/bevoelkerung.assetdetail.18845637.html.

Carraça, E., Encantado, J., Battista, F., Beaulieu, K., Blundell, J., Busetto, L., van Baak, M., Dicker, D., Ermolao, A., & Farpour-Lambert, N. (2021). Effective behavior change techniques to promote physical activity in adults with overweight or obesity: A systematic review and meta-analysis. *Obesity Reviews, 22*(S4), e13258. https://doi.org/10.1111/obr.13258.

Deci, E. L., & Ryan, R. M. (1985). The general causality orientations scale: Self-determination in personality. *Journal of Research in Personality, 19*(2), 109–134. https://doi.org/10.1016/0092-6566(85)90023-6.

DeSmet, A., Van Ryckeghem, D., Compernolle, S., Baranowski, T., Thompson, D., Crombez, G., Poels, K., Van Lippevelde, W., Bastiaensens, S., & Van Cleemput, K. (2014). A meta-analysis of serious digital games for healthy lifestyle promotion. *Preventive Medicine, 69,* 95–107. https://doi.org/10.1016/j.ypmed.2014.08.026.

Graesser, A., Chipman, P., & Leeming, F. (2009). Deep learning and emotion in serious games. In U. Ritterfeld, M. Cody, & P. Vorderer (Hrsg.), *Serious games: Mechanisms and effects* (S. 83–102). Routledge.

Hagger, M. S., Hankonen, N. E., & Ryan, R. M. (2020). Changing behavior using self-determination theory. In M. S. Hagger, L. D. Cameron, K. Hamilton, N. Hankonen, & T. Lintunen (Hrsg.), *The handbook of behavior change* (S. 104–119). Cambridge University Press. https://doi.org/10.1017/9781108677318.008.

Hennessy, E. A., Johnson, B. T., Acabchuk, R. L., McCloskey, K., & Stewart-James, J. (2020). Self-regulation mechanisms in health behavior change: A systematic meta-review of meta-analyses, 2006–2017. *Health Psychology Review, 14*(1), 6–42. https://doi.org/10.1080/17437199.2019.1679654.

Michie, S., Richardson, M., Johnston, M., Abraham, C., Francis, J., Hardeman, W., Eccles, M. P., Cane, J., & Wood, C. E. (2013). The behavior change technique taxonomy (v1) of 93 hierarchically clustered techniques: Building an international consensus for the reporting of behavior change interventions. *Annals of Behavioral Medicine, 46*(1), 81–95. https://doi.org/10.1007/s12160-013-9486-6.

Ng, J. Y. Y., Ntoumanis, N., Thøgersen-Ntoumani, C., Deci, E. L., Ryan, R. M., Duda, J. L., & Williams, G. C. (2012). Self-determination theory applied to health contexts: A meta-analysis. *Perspectives on Psychological Science, 7*(4), 325–340. https://doi.org/10.1177/1745691612447309.

Ryan, R. M., Deci, E. L., Vansteenkiste, M., & Soenens, B. (2021). Building a science of motivated persons: Self-determination theory's empirical approach to human experience and the regulation of behavior. *Motivation Science, 7*(2), 97–110. https://doi.org/10.1037/mot0000194.

Ryan, R., Patrick, H., Deci, E., & Williams, G. (2007). Facilitating health behavior change and its maintenance: Interventions based on self-determination theory. *The European Health Psychologist, 10*(1), 2–5.

Samdal, G. B., Eide, G. E., Barth, T., Williams, G., & Meland, E. (2017). Effective behaviour change techniques for physical activity and healthy eating in overweight and obese adults; systematic review and meta-regression analyses. *International Journal of Behavioral Nutrition and Physical Activity, 14*(1), 42. https://doi.org/10.1186/s12966-017-0494-y.

Sharpe, E. E., Karasouli, E., & Meyer, C. (2017). Examining factors of engagement with digital interventions for weight management: Rapid review. *JMIR Research Protocols, 6*(10), e205. https://doi.org/10.2196/resprot.6059.

Smit, E. S., & Bol, N. (2020). From self-reliers to expert-dependents: Identifying classes based on health-related need for autonomy and need for external control among mobile users. *Media Psychology, 23*(3), 391–414. https://doi.org/10.1080/15213269.2019.1604235.

van Vugt, M., de Wit, M., Cleijne, W. H., & Snoek, F. J. (2013). Use of behavioral change techniques in web-based self-management programs for type 2 diabetes patients: Systematic review. *Journal of Medical Internet Research, 15*(12), e279. https://doi.org/10.2196/jmir.2800.

Effectiveness of the Use of Digital Measures

6

Contents

Abstract

This chapter summarizes the approach and results of a study on the effectiveness of using different digital measures on measurable medical parameters. The study is based on field data collected with a digital health app. It shows that the use of digital services is associated with a positive development in weight-loss. In particular, it was demonstrated that there is a statistically significant correlation between the use of digital self-monitoring (biomarker tracking) and a reduction in weight.

Various studies have provided evidence that digital measures as implementation of behavior change techniques (BCTs) to promote a a healthy lifestyle effectively lead to successful behavior change. In the context of the present study, the effect of three digital

A. Schäfer et al., *Maintaining a Healthy Lifestyle*,
https://doi.org/10.1007/978-3-662-69460-2_6

measures on objectively measurable behavioral variables and medical parameters was examined in a real implementation context. The implementation context is a digital application that supports its users in changing their lifestyle towards a healthy diet and more exercise.

6.1   Initial Situation and Questions

The present study focused on the following three digital measures: 1) Biomarker tracking, 2) Automated coaching, and 3) Interaction with the ecosystem.

Biomarker Tracking corresponds to the behavior change technique of self-monitoring of results (behavior change technique 2.4 according to the classification by Michie et al. (2013), see also Sect. 2.2). As part of the biomarker tracking measure, users record various relevant biomarkers (e.g., weight or blood pressure) on the digital app. The functionality of the app facilitates monitoring. Furthermore, users receive feedback on their current status based on this. The implementation is shown in Fig. 6.1.

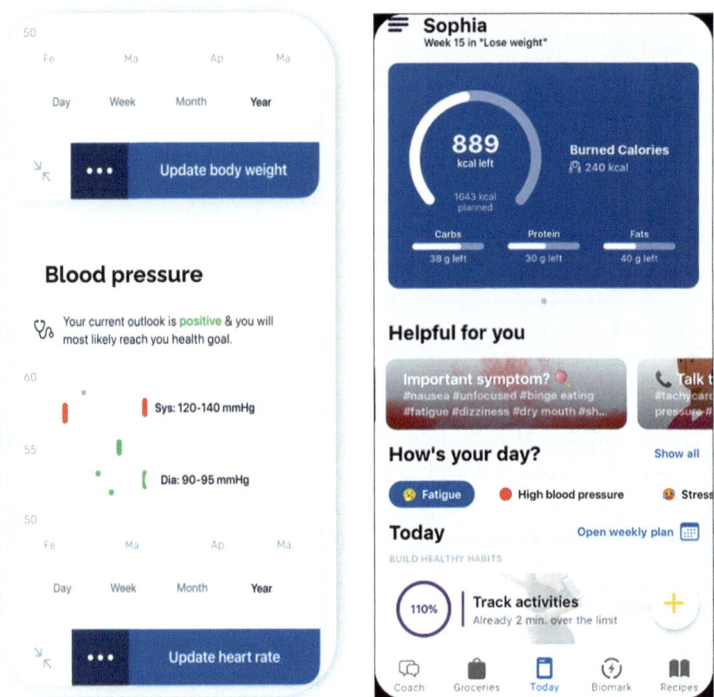

Fig. 6.1   Example of biomarker tracking. (Image courtesy of: Uplyfe.io)

The measure *Automated Coaching* corresponds to the behavior change technique "Instruction for behavior execution" (behavior change technique 4.1 according to the classification by Michie et al. (2013)). Based on the tracking, users automatically receive practical tips on how to deal with challenges, setbacks, and problems related to behaviors that are relevant for behavior change. An example is shown in Fig. 6.2.

The *Interaction with the Ecosystem* is a measure that can be associated with restructuring the environment behavior change techniques: The conditions are changed by connecting with other digital apps (e.g., step counters, nutrition apps, etc.) (behavior change technique 12.1 according to the classification by Michie et al. (2013)). This restructuring

Fig. 6.2 Example of automated coaching. (Image courtesy of: Uplyfe.io)

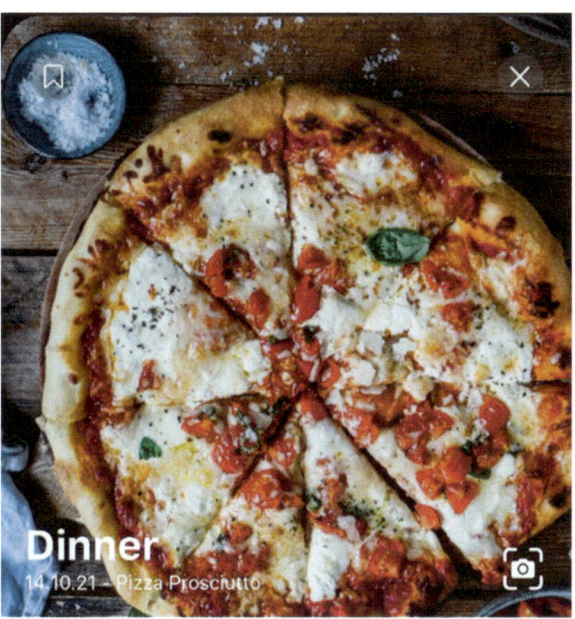

Dinner
14.10.21 – Pizza Prosciutto

 Pizza Prosciutto
1 Pizza

754 kcal

 Acceptable food choice but you can do better.

Your nutrition spotlight
More fiber please! They are important for your digestion and at the same time prolong your feeling of satiety. Next time, make sure you eat enough fruit, vegetables and wholemeal products.
Sophia | Uplyfe nutrition coach

of the context changes the behavior context in such a way that the desired behavior is facilitated. An example is shown in Fig. 6.3.

The effect is examined both at the level of acceptance (usage), at the behavioral level (physical activity), and at the level of medical measurements (weight, blood sugar level, and blood pressure).

Fig. 6.3 Example of interaction with the ecosystem. (Image courtesy of: Uplyfe.io)

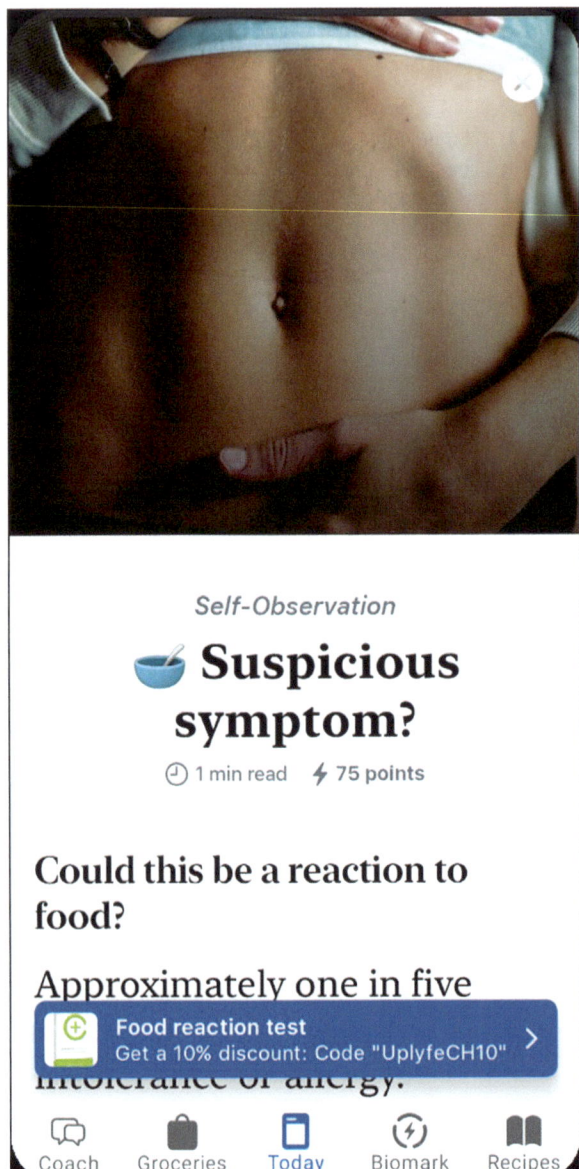

The study pursued the goal of answering the following research questions:

1. How frequently were the digital measures used by the users of the health apps?
   a) How frequently was the biomarker tracking used?
   b) How frequently was the automated coaching used?
   c) How frequently were interactions with the ecosystem used?
2. To what extent did the use of digital measures influencethe behavior of users?
   a) How does the use of biomarker tracking affect physical activity?
   b) How does the use of automated coaching affect physical activity?
   c) How does interaction with the ecosystem affect physical activity?
3. What effect does the use of digital measures have on medical indicators of lifestyle change (weight, blood sugar level, and blood pressure)?
   a) How does the use of biomarker tracking affect medical indicators?
   b) How does the use of automated coaching affect medical indicators?
   c) How does interaction with the ecosystem affect medical indicators?

To answer the research questions, usage data from the health app were evaluated. The following explains the procedure and subsequently presents and discusses the results.

6.2   Procedure for Measuring the Effectiveness of Digital Measures

The following describes the procedure for measuring the effectiveness of digital measures. After describing the data basis, the description of the sample and the procedure within the analysis follows.

6.2.1   Data Extraction and Data Basis

Usage data from the health app were extracted for the analysis. Data from a period of four months were used (March 2021 to June 2021). Only data from users that were active throughout the entire determined period of time was included. The variables that were considered for the data extraction are shown in Table 6.1.

The preparation and anonymization of the data were carried out by the data controllers of the health app. Only data relevant to answering the research question were extracted. Irrelevant information such as timestamps, personal data, IP addresses, etc. were deleted from the dataset, so that no conclusions about individual persons can be drawn from the data. The use of this data for the described research purpose is in accordance with Swiss data protection regulations and the data protection regulation of the health app, which the users have agreed to.

Table 6.1 Variables for Data Extraction

Category	Measures	Units/Measurements
Monitoring	Biomarker Tracking	Total usage over the entire period
Instruction for Behavior Execution	Automated Coachings	Total usage over the entire period
Change of Conditions	Interactions in the Ecosystem	Total usage over the entire period
Physical activity	Number of Steps	Number of steps per day at measurement time T_0 (start point of data selection) and measurement time T_1 (4 months after start point of data selection)
Weight	Body Weight	Kilograms of body weight to one decimal place at time T_0 (start point of data selection) and time T_1 (4 months after start point of data selection)
Blood Pressure	Diastolic and Systolic Blood Pressure	Blood pressure at time T_0 (start point of data selection) and time T_1 (4 months after start point of data selection)
Blood Sugar	Blood Sugar Levels	Blood sugar at time T_0 (start point of data selection) and time T_1 (4 months after start point of data selection)
Age		Years
Gender		Male/Female

6.2.2   Sample

From the entire data base of the users of the health app, the data of 956 users met the above conditions. For the analysis, data from 100 users were randomly selected from this dataset. In this randomly selected sample, 60 % of the individuals were women and 40 % were men. The age ranged from 23 to 72 years with an average of 48 years and a standard deviation of around 15 years.

6.2.3   Analysis

For the analysis of the data, differential values were formed for all effect variables (values T_0 minus T_1). The percentage weight change (relative to the initial weight) was additionally used to measure the effect on body weight. The data was analyzed using the statistical program SPSS Version 16. Only descriptive analyses (frequencies and correlations) were carried out.

6.3   Results

This section presents and summarizes the results from the descriptive analyses.

6.3.1   Usage Frequencies

The average usage frequencies of the three selected digital measures over the mentioned period are shown in Table 6.2. The biomarker tracking with an average of around 6700 uses was used very frequently overall. On average, users used this application about 55 times a day. It should be noted that 25 % of the users used the application only once.

Automated coachings are used much less frequently. Over the entire period, these were used on average only about six times. Here, 11 % of the users never used this application. A similar picture emerges with regard to the interactions in the ecosystem with a mean of 1.6 uses over the entire period and a proportion of 35 % who never used the application.

6.3.2   Correlations between the Frequency of use and Physical Activity

The descriptive analysis of the number of steps shows an increase in the number of steps taken by users over the examined period of four months: On average, users took around 1600 more steps per day. The standard deviation is around 1900 steps. The mean values range between minus 2000 steps and plus 6000 steps.

Table 6.2   Overview of the usage frequencies of the digital measures (mean values, standard deviation, minimum and maximum); $n = 100$

	Mean	Standard Deviation	Minimum	Maximum
Biomarker Tracking	6689	5478	1	16.716
Automated Coachings	5.9	4.5	0	16
Interactions in the Ecosystem	1.6	1.7	0	7

The analysis of the correlations shows that there are statistically relevant relationships between the differentill values of the number of steps and the use of biomarker tracking as well as automated coaching (see Table 6.3): The more frequently the digital applications are used, the greater the increase in the number of steps that users took on average per day. No statistically relevant correlation was found, however, between interactions in the ecosystem and the number of steps.

6.3.3   Correlations between the Frequency of use of Measures and the Medical Parameters Weight, Blood Pressure, and Blood Sugar

The descriptive analyses of the medical measurements show the development of blood pressure, blood sugar, and weight over a period of four months. The blood sugar level slightly increased for the examined period. When interpreting, it should be considered that data on blood sugar levels are only available for 45 % of the sample. This is because blood sugar levels are only known for users who suffer from diabetes or the metabolic syndrome.

The descriptive analysis of the development of blood pressure shows that the blood pressure values hardly changed over the period. When interpreting the values, it should be considered that data on blood pressure values are only available for 85 % of the sample.

The descriptive analyses of weight change reveal that the body weight of the subjects has reduced on average by 4 %. This corresponds to an average loss of five kilograms of body weight of the users.

The descriptive evaluations based on correlations show various statistically relevant relationships between the frequency of use of digital applications and medical measurement values (see Table 6.4).

For the use of biomarker tracking, a statistically significant positive correlation with blood sugar levels was found. This is an unfavorable outcome in terms of health. The negative correlation between biomarker tracking and relative weight loss, on the other

Table 6.3 Correlations of usage frequency with the difference values of number of steps (n = sample size)

Effect		Biomarker Tracking	Coachings	Interactions in the Ecosystem
	n	100	100	100
Difference values steps	Correlation according to Pearson	.299**	.202*	0.142

*The correlation is significant at the 0.05 level (2-tailed)
**The correlation is significant at the 0.01 level (2-tailed)

Table 6.4 Correlations of usage frequency with the difference values of medical values (n = sample size)

Effect		Biomarker Tracking	Coachings	Interactions in the Ecosystem
Difference value blood sugar	Correlation according to Pearson	,303*	−0,064	0,118
	n	45	45	45
Difference values blood pressure (systolic)	Correlation according to Pearson	−0,051	−0,015	−0.190
	n	85	85	85
Difference values blood pressure (diastolic)	Correlation according to Pearson	−0,192	−,230*	−0,061
	n	85	85	85
Relative difference values weight	Correlation according to Pearson	−,234*	−,313**	−,253*
	n	100	100	100

*The correlation is significant at the level of 0.05 (2-sided)
**The correlation is significant at the level of 0.01 (2-sided)

hand, shows the desired development: the more frequently biomarker tracking was used, the greater was the relative weight loss. No correlation was found between the use of biomarker tracking and blood pressure values.

The results show a statistically relevant negative correlation between the use of automated coaching and diastolic blood pressure as well as relative weight loss. These are desired outcomes: The more frequently automated coaching was used, the greater the reduction in blood pressure and weight. No correlation could be found between the coaching and physical activity (number of steps) or systolic blood pressure.

Between the interactions in the ecosystem and the various medical measurements, a significant correlation only results in relation to the relative weight change. As with the other digital applications, the data suggest that more frequent use is associated with a greaterweight reduction. There is no correlation between the interactions in the ecosystem and blood sugar and blood pressure values.

6.4 Conclusion

The three examined digital measures are used by users at different frequencies. Even though different usage frequencies are to be expected due to the nature of the offers, the analyses show that tracking as self-monitoring enjoys the greatest acceptance. More complex forms of support such as information or interactions within the health care ecosystem are only seldomly used.

Overall, the use of the selected digital measures shows a statistically relevant correlation with some of the behavioural and health related outcomes. The more frequently automated coaching (i.e., instructions for behavior execution) is used, the greater the weight loss, the more favorable the blood pressure development, and the increase in physical activity. The use of biomarker tracking is associated with two aspects of a healthy lifestyle. There is a positive correlation with physical activity and a negative correlation with weight development. In terms of interaction with the ecosystem, only a significant effect in terms of weight reduction is measured. There is no statistically relevant correlation with the medical target values of blood sugar and blood pressure.

When interpreting the results, limitations must be taken into account: The effect measurement is based on descriptive analyses of existing app usage data. Correlational relationships are always only an indication of possible causal relationships. It is also not an experimental setting in which the outcomes in a treatment group are compared with the outcomes in a control group. Therefore, it cannot be ruled out that other, additional factors are responsible for the positive outcomes towards a healthy lifestyle. This disadvantage is offset by the advantage of a field study with high ecological validity: The data were collected in the field and show effects among users.

These results thus form the basis for further studies on the causal relationships between measures and medical health related outcomes. They provide an evicence based foundation for the recommendation to promote the use of digital measures such as biomarker tracking or coaching.

References

Michie, S., Richardson, M., Johnston, M., Abraham, C., Francis, J., Hardeman, W., Eccles, M. P., Cane, J., & Wood, C. E. (2013). The behavior change technique taxonomy (v1) of 93 hierarchically clustered techniques: Building an international consensus for the reporting of behavior change interventions. *Annals of Behavioral Medicine, 46*(1), 81–95. https://doi.org/10.1007/s12160-013-9486-6.

Analysis of the Customer Journey in the Health Ecosystem

Contents

Abstract

This chapter is dedicated to the validation of the Customer Journey in the maintenance stage. Touchpoints in the health ecosystem with which those affected interact during the maintenance stage, are of interes here, as well as the importance of
self-management. In-depth interviews with 20 individuals who have successfully
changed their lifestyle for at least six months serve as the data basis. This shows that
the maintenance stage is an iterative process that always starts with the activity "setting goal(s)". For those affected, sticking to a healthy lifestyle does not happen "automatically", but they set themselves new adapted goals. The relevant touchpoints are
individuals, organizations, and digital tools from the health ecosystem, with the latter
gaining in importance. Self-management plays a decisive role in living a healthy life
in the long term. Digital measures can significantly support the degree of autonomy of
those affected.

In the maintenance stage, the goal is to establish a new habit, that is, to maintain a healthy lifestyle. How do those affected cope with the fact that old behaviors still pose a temptation, that there are challenges to overcome (e.g., when eating out), and that they need to deal with not being successful? The following research questions should therefore be answered by means of a qualitative impact study:

1. What activities make up the overarching consumer journey of the maintenance stage and what customer journeys can be derived from it?
2. How do those affected perceive the consumer journey and what emotions do they experience during the activities?
3. What communication channels do those affected use today and in the future during the consumer journey?
4. Which ecosystem partners are relevant today and in the future for the respective activities along the consumer journey?
5. What role does self-management play in the maintenance stage?

Answers to research questions 1 to 3 are summarized in Sect. 7.2. Section 7.3 addresses the fourth research question and Sect. 7.4 addresses the fifth research question. A summarizing conclusion of the findings is drawn in Sect. 7.5.

7.1　　Procedure and Methodology

The present study applies a phenomenological research methodology, which relies particularly on interpretative and hermeneutic approaches (Thompson et al., 1989). The aim of this research method is to uncover essential, unchangeable characteristics of conscious, immediate experiences (Goulding, 2005). To understand the maintenance phase in the present study, the subjective experiences of those affected must be understood and localised in their lifeworld. In terms of the research process, this means using the views and experiences of those affected as data sources. This presupposes that the subjective perspective of those affected is considered as "fact". Furthermore participants in the study are only those who have had the experience under investigation. The sampling is therefore targeted and prescribed from the outset (Goulding, 2005). Accordingly, 20 people were interviewed who had changed their lifestyle for health reasons (diabetes, obesity, high blood pressure, heart problems, etc.) at least six months ago and are in the maintenance phase. The guideline-based interviews were not conducted in person due to the Corona pandemic situation, but with the help of the video conferencing software Zoom. This ensured that the interviewer and interviewees could see each other. Visual elements (e.g., showing the activities of a consumer journey) were used for the interviews via virtual online collaboration tools, including Miro boards (RealtimeBoard Inc. dba Miro, n. d.).

The interviews, that lasted approximately 60 minutes, were recorded and then transcribed in MAXQDA. For data interpretation, two researchers independently read the interview transcripts completely and first obtained a general overview. Subsequently, they looked for patterns and differences in the transcripts. This interpretation strategy recommends expanding the analyses to include a broader spectrum of considerations and ultimately to arrive at a holistic interpretation. This means that the researchers' interpretations always include considerations from the theoretical literature (Goulding, 2005).

The sample of 20 people consists of eleven women and nine men who were recruited through a market research institute. The age of the respondents ranges from 22 to 70 years, with the average age of just over 48.6 years being slightly above the average of the Swiss population (42.6 years, Federal Statistical Office, 2021). At the time of the study (November to December 2020), the respondents had changed their lifestyle for health reasons such as obesity (eight mentions) and type II diabetes (seven mentions) at least six months ago and were thus in the maintenance stage of lifestyle change.

7.2   Consumer Journey and Customer Journeys of the Maintenance Stage

7.2.1   Activities in the Consumer Journey of the Maintenance Stage and in the Customer Journeys Exercise and Nutrition

Answer to research question 1: What activities make up the overarching consumer journey of the maintenance phase and what customer journeys can be derived from it?

In accordance with the structuring of the Customer Journey by Becker et al. (2020), the present study examined, within the context of the *Consumer Journey*, the structure of the maintenance stage for those affected, i.e., what activities they go through to maintain a healthy lifestyle. The Consumer Journey in the maintenance phase consists of the activities "setting goals/planning implementation", "implementing activities", "checking progress", "receiving feedback" and "receiving reward" (see Fig. 7.1).

The interviews were used to validate that the activities "setting goals/planning implementation", "implementing activities", "checking progress" are all carried out by those affected in the maintenance stage. This stage therefore involves a subordinate process that is similar to the overall process of behavior change according to the stage model (see Sect. 2.1.1).

Interviewee 9 expressed it as follows: *"The first three (activities) are the foundation, they are really necessary". "Checking progress"* implies for some affected people that they receive feedback on the status of goal achievement. For others affected, "receiving feedback" is a separate fourth step, e.g., in the form of body fat measurements or feedback from friends. The activity "receiving reward" is not, rather not or no longer relevant for 12 interviewees. Only for five respondents is this activity important, leading to the assumption that there is a shortened version of the Consumer Journey in the maintanance

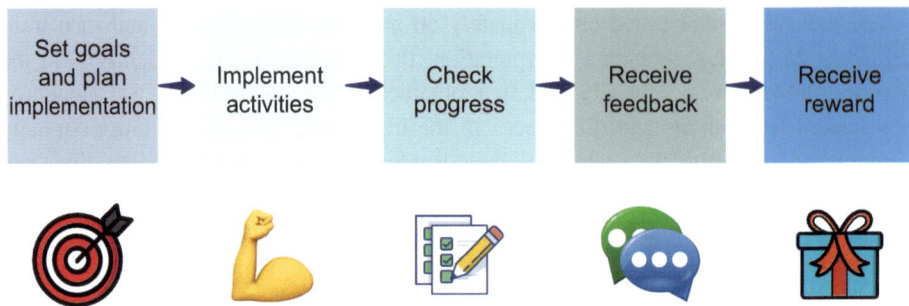

Fig. 7.1 Consumer Journey of the maintenance stage

stage. If the activity "receiving reward" is not relevant, it is justified as follows: *"Reward for me is actually when I have reached the goal. That is reward enough"* (Interview 9). If rewards play a role, they can take a material form: *"…you might buy a T-shirt that you didn't dare to wear before because it accentuates the is figure-hugging"* (Interview 18). Those affected reward themselves either independently of others or in interaction with others, e.g. shopping for clothes together or receiving a compliment. *"When I want to buy something new to wear, my girlfriend comes with me as a good advisor. If it's with the partner, then it's usually going out for a nice meal "* (Interview 18).

If the activities listed in Fig. 7.1 are categorised in the Consumer Journey according to different "stages", i.e., phases (Homburg et al., 2017), then the activity "setting goals and planning implementation" belongs to the "pre-core stage", while "implementing activities" represents the main phase or "core stage" and the last three activities "checking progress" as well as optionally "receiving feedback" and "receiving reward" can be attributed to the "post-core stage".

A key finding is that the Consumer Journey for the maintenance stage is an iterative process: *"You have to go through these steps over and over again with new goals, exactly. Adjust the goals a bit to the situation"* (Interview 5). Those affected therefore repeatedly go through the subordinate process of behavior change. This is an important finding for those affected, because they obviously cannot rely on the fact that a healthy lifestyle will "automatically" come about and remain sustainable. Rather, "sticking with it" is an active process that repeatedly requires those affected to set new and adapted goals and plan activities, implement them, check progress and subsequently optionally obtain feedback and receive a reward from themselves or third parties.

The interviews reveal that the consumer journey "maintaining a healthy lifestyle" includes two different customer journeys, which relate to nutrition and exercise (see Fig. 7.2). One customer journey pursues the objective of a healthy, fat-reduced, and balanced diet. The other customer journey aims for sufficient exercise. While the activities described above "setting goals/planning implementation", "implementing activities", "checking progress", "receiving feedback", and "receiving rewards" are the same for

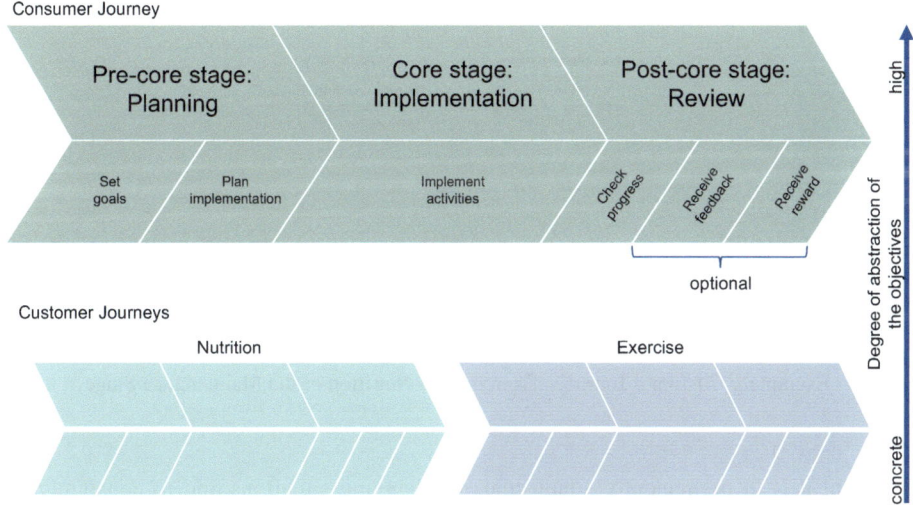

Fig. 7.2   Consumer Journey and Customer Journeys of the Maintenance Stage

both customer journeys, they differ in the touchpoints. In the customer journey for nutrition, nutritionists are important touchpoints in the pre-core stage and the post-core stage, while in the customer journey for exercise, gyms or sports clubs often play a central role in the core stage. The interviewees confirm that the overarching goal of a sustainably healthy lifestyle can only be achieved if both the nutrition and exercise customer journeys are consistently pursued. Only one person was of the opinion that exercise plays a subordinate role. This result is in line with various studies, according to which a combination of measures from the areas of nutrition and exercise bring sustainable success (e.g., The Diabetes Prevention Program Research Group, 2002).

In Fig. 7.2, the degree of abstraction of the goals is shown on the right. The overarching goal of the consumer journey is abstract and not operationalized. At the level of the respective customer journeys nutrition and exercise, the interviewees confirm that they usually formulate their goals concretely and their implementation is usually measurable. For example, interviewee 16 defines his daily exercise goal: *"1,000 steps in one go, then I am physically exhausted, but it builds me up"*. The exemplary implementation (see Fig. 7.3) shows how closely exercise and nutrition can be linked: *"I go to the market twice a week, then I also get exercise and I always buy healthy things and so I have exercise and have shopped healthily"* (Interview 16). The exercise is checked using a pedometer and a heart rate monitor. In terms of nutrition, interviewee 16 pays close attention to consuming fresh products. With the help of a nutritionist who supported him in the transition phase, he was able to acquire sufficient knowledge to be able to carry out the monitoring in a cognitive information processing process. The following quote illustrates how

Exemplary customer journey movement

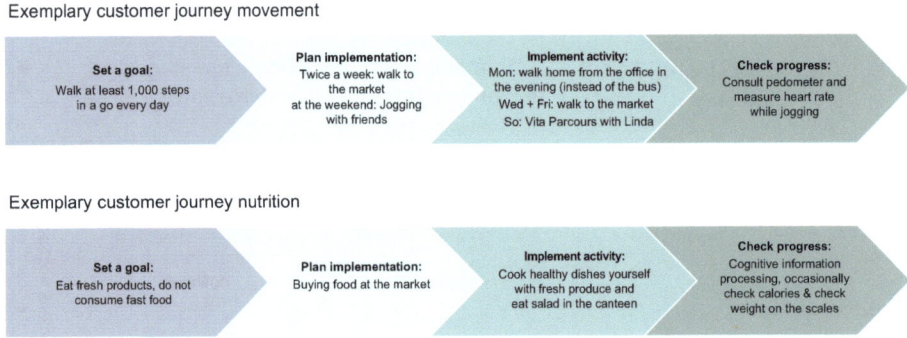

Exemplary customer journey nutrition

Fig. 7.3 Exemplary Customer Journeys Exercise and Nutrition of the Maintenance Stage

important it is to permanently adapt goals to changing situations and to constantly set new goals: *"And when you have reached the first goals, then you look forward to the new goal setting."* (Interview 11).

7.2.2 Emotions During the Consumer Journey

Answering research question 2: How do those affected perceive the consumer journey, what emotions do they feel during the activities?

Emotions modify or dominate customer behavior from a certain intensity. Emotions are positive or negative because from the customer's perspective, they help to achieve goals better or worse, or not at all. The interviewees were asked to assess their emotions along the consumer journey. On a Likert scale from 1 to 5 (1 = very dissatisfied; 5 = very satisfied), the values were overall in the upper, satisfactory range (see Fig. 7.4). All activities are associated with positive emotions: While "setting goals and planning implementation" and "checking progress" reached an average of 3.8 each, "implementing activities" and "reward" were rated 4.5, slightly better than "receiving feedback" (4.4). It shows that the activities associated with implementing a healthy lifestyle are positively connoted. This is also an important finding that can be used to motivate those affected.

Even though those affected generally associate the consumer journey with positive emotions, they report challenges that can be summarised into clusters. It is striking that the interviewees often refer to the challenges of the customer journey of healthy eating, whereas going through the customer journey of exercise apparently poses less difficulty. Especially when perceived stagnation occurs, motivation decreases and there is a risk of deviating from the consistent pursuit of the consumer journey: *"Then you see no result and self-doubt arises again. Surely once a month this happens"* (Interview 9). Various forms of stress (e.g., high workload, grief) or simply "deviating from everyday life"

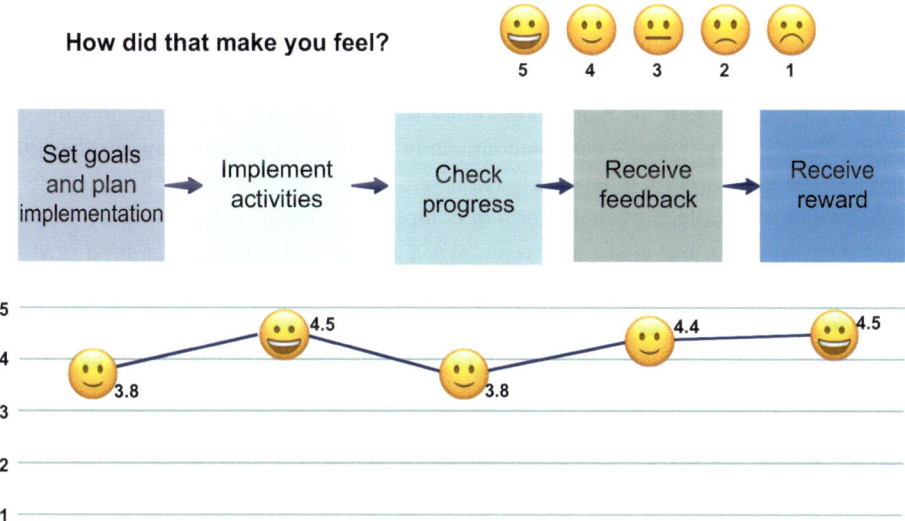

Fig. 7.4 Emotion curve of those affected during the consumer journey

(Interview 8) are mentioned as challenges. Social and cultural aspects of eating also pose a challenge for those affected: Not only when eating with other family members (*"… and the partner just eats completely different things,"* Interview 1), but also with friends, there are obstacles to overcome: *"Being invited to friends, that's a challenge, e.g., eating fondue. Declining an invitation"* (Interview 16). This also applies to eating out with friends: *"When I have to go out to eat in a group, for example, it's difficult because then I have to make sure I don't eat things that are bad for cholesterol"* (Interview 19). The product presentation in retail stores, e.g., the seasonal extra placement of sweets or the necessity to eat healthy on the go, are also mentioned as challenges. Finally, the interviewees state that the communication of a healthy lifestyle is not a matter of course. Apparently, it is perceived negatively that one has to explain oneself.

Those affected develop strategies to deal with these challenges. Self-management and mindfulness are very important. For example, Interviewee 1 reports: *"…because I slowly discover mechanisms for myself that work both in the restaurant and with friends. It's also a process, because at the beginning, when you've outed yourself to your social environment that you've made a different decision for yourself, the reactions are also special. You have to learn to deal with it."* Interviewee 10 explains, for example, that he practices mental training in the form of yoga in order to not feel pressured. In summary, it can be stated that challenges occur partly in the planning phase, but as expected more often in the implementation phase. Familiy members and friends provide important support in mastering challenges. Self-management of those affected is also very important for successful handling of challenges. This is explained in detail in Sect. 7.4.

Moments of success obviously contribute to the positive course of the emotion curve. These occur especially when "checking progress" and during feedback. "Checking progress" per se is a neutral activity, monitoring progress could even lead to unpleasant emotions, for example if the scale shows more weight. However, it is noticeable that the activity "checking progress" was predominantly positively connoted among the interviewees. The same applies to feedback. However, it is not only important to receive feedback from other people, e.g., in the form of compliments, but it is also important to share one's own joy about the goals achieved: *"When I swam a kilometer, I showed it to my family, on my watch. And they were happy for me because I had wanted to do that for a long time … I do share that, … face-to-face, so I can see how they are happy"* (Interview 14). Successes are most likely shared with friends, followed by the doctor and family.

7.2.3   Use of Communication Channels During the Consumer Journey

Answering research question 3: Which communication channels do those affected use today and in the future during the consumer journey?

For communication at the touchpoints, the affected individuals use various channels: Personal contact (face-to-face), telephone, and app/chat function/email. According to the study results, face- to -face is the most important channel. Often, those affected have a central person of trust for lifestyle changes with whom they exchange information. Half of the respondents identify the doctor as the central person of trust, six respondents mention the nutritionist. Face-to-face dominates these touchpoints; only when a certain level of trust has been built up, digital channels are mentioned or are even preferred. *"So I can imagine some online support, because I know the person… I can imagine it in terms of the type, but [it does] not have the same quality and alone, I can't imagine it. It would always have to be in combination with face-to-face"* (Interview 11). According to the interviewees, the Corona pandemic has contributed to a stronger use of digital channels (telephone, app, chat) and these will likely remain significant in the future.

7.3   Relevance of Partners from the Health Ecosystem

Answering research question 4: Which ecosystem partners (touchpoints) are relevant today and in the future for the respective activities along the consumer journey?

Those affected interact with touchpoints during their customer journey. These touchpoints are either human actors of the healthcare ecosystem or impersonal touchpoints, such as an app or website. The touchpoints can be divided into three categories: (1) People from the social environment of those affected, such as partners, family members, friends, and people in similar situations. In Transformative Service Research (TSR) they all belong to the micro level(see Fig. 1.1, Sect. 1.3); (2) Health service providers including doctors, physiotherapists, and nutritionists, health insurance companies, pharmacies, sports clubs, fitness studios; they belong to the meso level. (3) Technical aids, e.g. mobile devices, scales, health apps, pedometers, and calorie counters. The technical aids are usually offered by representatives or organizations of the meso level. However, since they support those affected in checking progress and/or obtaining feedback and take on the function of the "extended self" (see also explanations below), they belong to the micro level in the context of the study. No study participant had direct contact with representatives of the macro level, i.e. cantonal or national health authorities, i.e. they do not function as a direct touchpoint. Nevertheless, these macro-level organizations influence indirectly those affected.

To determine the relevance of the touchpoints on the consumer journey, all previously relevant touchpoints as well as additional desired touchpoints per activity of the consumer journey were surveyed in the interviews. The determined relevance of the touchpoints is based on the number of mentions across all interviews. The maximum value of the mention results from the multiplication of the number of interviews (20) and the number of activities (5) and is therefore 100. In this way, the actual situation (see Fig. 7.5) as well as the desired situation (target) (see Fig. 7.6) can be visualised.

The most frequently mentioned touchpoint in the consumer journey is the technical tool (55 mentions), followed by doctor (45 mentions), friends (31 mentions), partner (27 mentions), nutrisionist (26 mentions), club/fitness studio (19 mentions), family (18 mentions), and people in similar situations (13 mentions). Health insurance companies and

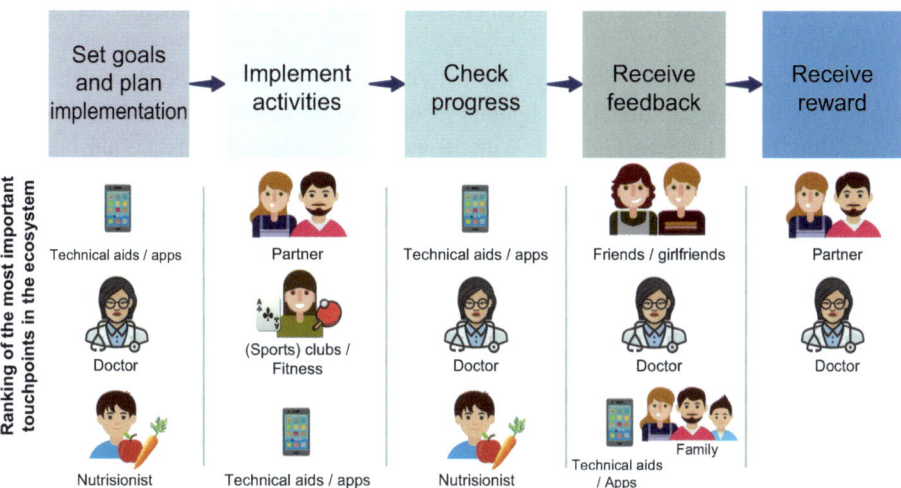

Fig. 7.5 Main touchpoints (ACTUAL) Consumer Journey

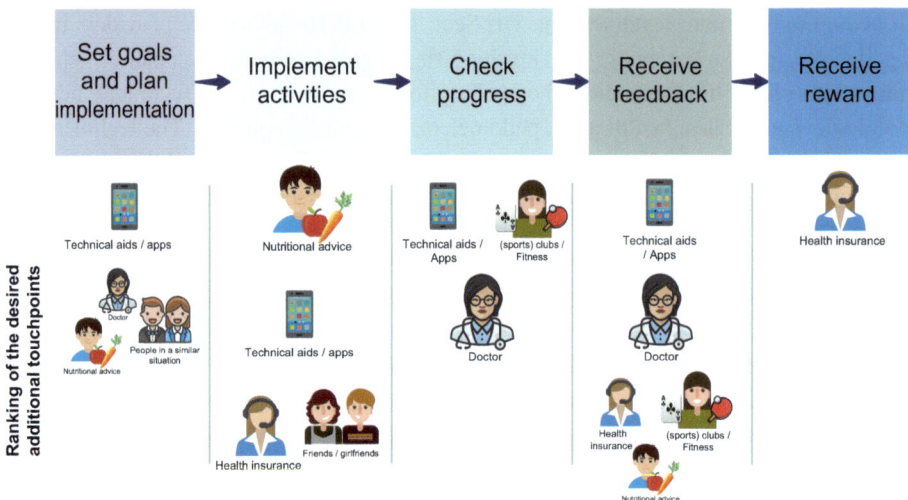

Reading example: In the "Implement activities" step, nutritional advice was mentioned most frequently, followed by technical aids and health insurance and friends.

Fig. 7.6   Desired additional touchpoints (TARGET) Consumer Journey

pharmacies, on the other hand, play a very subordinate role. Fig. 7.5 shows that technical tools dominate especially in the activities "setting goals and planning implementation" and "checking progress". But also in implementation and feedback, those affected use them often. The high relevance of doctor as well as family and partner is consistent with the results of the quantitative impact study (Chap. 5). A central role is played by the affected persons themselves (patient-centeredness). This applies in particular for "implementing activities".

In the target consumer journey, the activities remain the same. However, those affected would like additional touchpoints in order to be better supported in "sticking to a healthy lifestyle" (see Fig. 7.6). With 18 mentions, technical tools are attributed an increase in importance, even though they already have a high relevance today. Those affected would also like more support from health service providers: nutritionist (14), doctor (12) health insurance (9), club/fitness studio (9) and pharmacy (1). The social environment could also provide better support: friends (8), partner (6), family (6), people in similar situations (6) are mentioned. Fig. 7.4 provides information on which phases of the consumer journey additional touchpoints would be helpful.

The health ecosystem is an open and dynamic system. This is evident, among other things, from the fact that there are a large number of new providers entering the lifestyle market. These are often companies that develop apps or digital offers. The importance of technical aids is expected to increase. This can be interpreted as a shift in the interaction line, especially in the activity "receiving feedback". An example illustrates this: While in the past the doctor monitored e.g., blood sugar level, and this was a "brand-owned" touchpoint of the service provider according to Lemon and Verhoef (2016), technical tools now allow those affected to perform the measurement themselves. The monitoring is thus "internalized" by them and the "brand-owned" touchpoint becomes a customer-owned touchpoint. The doctor is only involved in this activity of the consumer journey when deviations or emergencies occur. In this sense, technical tools can be considered as an Extended Self (in reference to Belk, 2013, p. 477). They not only provide those affected with a functional benefit (e.g., information about the blood sugar level), but also an emotional benefit (e.g., satisfaction) and thus also promote the individuality and self-determination of those affected.

7.4   The Role of Self-Management in the Maintenance Stage

Answer to research question 5: What role does self-management play in the maintenance stage?

The active role of those affected has already been discussed under the term "co-creation" in Chap. 3.1, The qualitative impact study therefore focussed on the question of of how strongly the adherence to a healthy lifestyle depends on those affected themselves or on others. To this end, the interviewees were asked to prioritise the responsibility for maintaining a healthy lifestyle on a scale from 1 (others are responsible) to 5 (I am responsible) (see Fig. 7.7). Almost all respondents positioned themselves on the scale between 4 and 5. The mean value was 4.7.

Those affected are aware that they play an active role in the maintenance stage: *"It's my health and if I mess it up, it's my own fault. It's also my responsibility to ask for help when I need it,"* (Interview 8). But that doesn't mean that ecosystem partners lose relevance. Rather, broad support from the environment can lead to those affected achieving a higher degree of autonomy.

The interviews revealed that those affected initiate co-creation activities themselves, which help them to better master the situation. Table 7.1 provides information about co-creation activities that are successfully used in the maintenance stage (McColl-Kennedy et al., 2012):

The results show a clear picture: The responsibility for behavioral change is attributed to the individual themselves. This understanding is related to the findings of

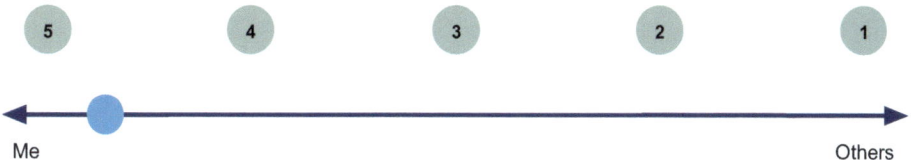

Fig. 7.7   Importance of self-management (scale: 5 = I am responsible; 1 = others are responsible)

Table 7.1 Co-creation activities

Co-creation activities in the maintenance phase	Examples	Quotes from the interviews
Cooperating	Receiving information from the service provider and adhering to the basics	*"I had a nutritional consultation, with a restriction on sugar, with exercise—I now do a lot of exercise."* Interview 18
Collating information	Sorting and organizing information, coping with simple everyday tasks	*"Yes, the [doctor] … says, I am one of the few patients who knows so well and keeps such meticulous records. And I can join in the conversation."* Interview 21
Combining complementary therapies	Use of alternative medicine, exercise, diet, yoga, meditation	*"In an emergency, meditation helps me."* Interview 1
Co-learning	Active search for and exchange of information from other sources	*"Literature, not necessarily nutritional advice but a lot of literature."* Interview 1
Connecting	Building and maintaining relationships	*"These contacts are very important to me. Especially when you reach a certain age. I am not becoming lonely, on the contrary, but such contacts are very important and you must not just say I have grown older and now simply have no more contacts, but maintain these. That motivates."* Interview 17

self-regulation in the strict sense (see Chap. 2). This also makes it clear that the ability to self-regulate as a personality trait is considered to be very important.

At the same time, the results explained in Table 7.1 show that those affected apply diverse self-management strategies that can beconsidered as co-creation activity. In implementation, self-regulation proves to be a skill that can be further developed with support within the ecosystem, i.e., support from outside and not just by the person themselves. A reference can also be made to the quantitative impact study (Chap. 5) at this point. This study also showed that those affected appreciate behavioral techniques that adress their own autonomy.

Overall, these results lead to the conclusion that services in the ecosystem should be designed to support the autonomy of those affected.

7.5   Conclusion

The consumer journey in the maintenance phase is an iterative process that begins with the activity "setting goal(s)". For those affected, the maintanance of a healthy lifestyle does not occur "automatically", but is facilitated by setting new and adapted goals. This means that those affected go through a subordinate process of behavior change again and again in the maintanance stage. While the activities "setting goals/planning implementation", "implementing activities" and "checking progress" are fixed components of the consumer journey and are repeatedly gone through, the activities "receiving feedback" and "receiving reward" are optional. At the level of the customer journey, where those affected pursue concrete goals, two relevant journeys could be identified: nutrition and exercise. These are linked, i.e., the maintenance of a healthy lifestyle is only successful if both the nutrition goals and the exercise goals are achieved. Even though those affected repeatedly face challenges in maintaining a healthy lifestyle, the emotional curve is overall assessed as positive. Especially the phase "implementing activities" evokes positive emotions. As expected, the importance of technical aids increases at the touchpoints. This is also due to the fact that technical aids allow those affected a higher degree of autonomy. Thus, checking progress can now be carried out by those affected themselves, whereas in the past they had to visit a doctor for certain monitoring checkups. However, this does not mean that technical aids replace human contact. Those affected desire more support from individuals and organizations at the meso-, but also at the micro level. They also see themselves as highly responsible for maintaining a healthy lifestyle. Digital support measures should therefore focus on goal setting and goal monitoring (checking progress) and support those affected in increasing their degree of autonomy.

References

Becker, L., Jaakkola, E., & Halinen, A. (2020). Toward a goal-oriented view of customer journeys. *Journal of Service Management, 31*(4), 767–790. https://doi.org/10.1108/JOSM-11-2019-0329,

Belk, R. W. (2013). Extended self in a digital world. *Journal of consumer research, 40*(3), 477–500.

Bundesamt für Statistik. (2021, September 30). Durchschnittsalter der ständigen Wohnbevölkerung nach Staatsangehörigkeitskategorie, Geschlecht und Kanton, 2010–2020—2010–2020 | Tabelle. Bundesamt für Statistik. https://www.bfs.admin.ch/bfs/de/home/statistiken/kataloge-daten-banken/tabellen.assetdetail.18845637.html,

Goulding, C. (2005). Grounded theory, ethnography and phenomenology: A comparative analysis of three qualitative strategies for marketing research. *European Journal of Marketing, 39*(3/4), 294–308. https://doi.org/10.1108/03090560510581782,

Homburg, C., Jozić, D., & Kuehnl, C. (2017). Customer experience management: Toward implementing an evolving marketing concept. *Journal of the Academy of Marketing Science, 45*(3), 377–401. https://doi.org/10.1007/s11747-015-0460-7,

Lemon, K. N., & Verhoef, P. C. (2016). Understanding customer experience throughout the customer journey. *Journal of Marketing, 80*(6), 69–96. https://doi.org/10.1509/jm.15.0420,

McColl-Kennedy, J. R., Vargo, S. L., Dagger, T. S., Sweeney, J. C., & van Kasteren, Y. (2012). Health care customer value cocreation practice styles. *Journal of Service Research, 15*(4), 370–389. https://doi.org/10.1177/1094670512442806,

RealtimeBoard Inc. dba Miro. (n. d.). Für Unternehmen ausgelegtes Online-Collaboration-Whiteboard. https://miro.com/, https://miro.com/de/enterprise/. Accessed 22. Dec. 2021.

The Diabetes Prevention Program Research Group. (2002). The Diabetes Prevention Program (DPP): Description of lifestyle intervention. *Diabetes Care, 25*(12), 2165–2171. https://doi.org/10.2337/diacare.25.12.2165,

Thompson, C. J., Locander, W. B., & Pollio, H. R. (1989). Putting consumer experience back into consumer research: The philosophy and method of existential-phenomenology. *Journal of Consumer Research, 16*(2), 133. https://doi.org/10.1086/209203,

The Role of Pharmacies within the Health Ecosystem

8

Contents

Abstract

The aim of the present study is to understand the current situation of pharmacies and drugstores within the health ecosystem and to comprehend the role they play in the maintenance phase of a lifestyle change. To this end, a best-practice analysis of consulting models and collaborations in the health ecosystem was conducted. The analysis is based on a literature review on challenges and potentials of pharmacies as well as six expert interviews with managers of pharmacies and drugstores, which belong to the distribution network of the research partner Dr. Bähler Dropa AG. The results suggest a new positioning of pharmacies and drugstores within the changing health ecosystem, which also takes into account interprofessionalism.

© The Author(s), under exclusive license to Springer-Verlag GmbH, DE, part of Springer Nature 2024
A. Schäfer et al., *Maintaining a Healthy Lifestyle*,
https://doi.org/10.1007/978-3-662-69460-2_8

8.1   Analysis of the Positioning of Pharmacies in Switzerland

Answering the research question: What role do pharmacies and drugstores play in the health ecosystem for a long-term lifestyle change?

One aspect of the present research project aims at investigating the roles of the various actors in the health ecosystem that they take on for a sustainable lifestyle change. These actors also include pharmacies, which according to the results of the quantitative impact study (Chap. 5) and the qualitative impact study (Chap. 7) are currently attributed a rather low importance in the ecosystem from the perspective of those affected. At the same time, pharmacies and drugstores are assumed to have a higher potential for accompanying towards a sustainable lifestyle change, hence they were considered separately in this last study of the research project. Initially, a literature search was conducted on the challenges and future potentials of pharmacies. The results of this research, along with expert interviews with pharmacists and drugstore employees, form the basis for a best-practice analysis. This provides a foundation for the development of consulting models and collaborations of pharmacies with other actors in the Swiss health ecosystem.

8.1.1   Opportunities and Challenges for the Swiss Pharmacy and Drugstore Market

In 2019, the Swiss Pharmacists' Association recorded 1806 pharmacies in Switzerland. This number has changed only slightly over the past ten years (pharmaSuisse, 2020). Among the service providers in the healthcare sector, pharmacies are perceived as neutral and easily accessible service providers, as they can be consulted outside the opening hours of doctor's offices and without prior appointment. The core business of pharmacies includes the dispensing of medications and other health-related products as well as the associated competent advice. In this way, pharmacies make a substantial contribution to basic medical care in Switzerland.

Increasingly, pharmacies are facing a difficult competitive situation. This is due, for example, to the peculiarity that in the majority of Swiss cantons (especially in German-speaking Switzerland), doctor's offices are allowed to dispense medications without the examination by a pharmacy (Fishman et al., 2018). This so-called self-dispensation directly affects the business area of pharmacies and can lead to increased competition between doctor's offices and pharmacies.

Recent trends, such as the advancing digitalization and the spread of online trade, are reflected in the form of pure online pharmacies and make the business of stationary pharmacies more difficult (Fitte & Teuteberg, 2019), especially in the area of low-consultation standard products (Frick & Schäfer, 2020). A look at the market in the USA suggests that competition could intensify here as well. Two factors are responsible for these developments: Firstly, so-called Retail Health Clinics at large retailers such as supermarket and drugstore chains (e.g. Walmart) offer a cheap standard range of medications and health services (Gerste, 2007). Secondly, digital health platforms are increasingly emerging, which serve as the first point of contact in the health system and connect service providers and customers in a very efficient way. An example of such a platform is Amazon Care (Amazon Care, n. d.). Currently, such offers are not yet available in Switzerland, as this market is strictly regulated (Fitte & Teuteberg, 2019), but there is clearly a trend towards digital and telemedical health offers. This is understandable from the perspective of cost carriers such as health insurance companies, but also from the perspective of service recipients themselves, as telemedical services are generally more cost-efficient than personal offers (Martin et al., 2018).

The increasing digitalization in the health sector also opens up opportunities for pharmacies in this country, if technological progress and a growing richness of data are used efficiently (Frick et al., 2020). These include, for example, health apps and wearables, i.e. body-worn technical devices that measure health data. Martin et al. (2018) see a possibility to strengthen the role of pharmacies in the health system. Due to their easy access, pharmacies offer good conditions for advising and disseminating new health technologies. A targeted data analysis by pharmacies can represent a significant added value for customers. This is in line with the recommendation made by Fitte and Teuteberg (2019) to strive for a technology-driven expansion of the service offer for local pharmacies, for example by pointing out apps and accompanying, competent advice. The authors see a specific need, among other things, in the area of disease prevention. However, models are still lacking for services, such as more intensive advice in the pharmacy, to be billed (Pfeifer, 2014).

In relation to the ecosystem approach described in Chap. 3, considerable potential is also predicted for pharmacies. In this context, the term ecosystem refers to the definition of a service ecosystem by Vargo and Lusch (2016). It is described as a self-adapting system of actors who pursue a common goal and share resources for this purpose. Consequently, a service is not provided by a single provider, but rather arises from individual, value-adding service parts of different actors, which in their entirety result in a service that is difficult to imitate (Leimeister, 2020). As a neutral and low-threshold contact within the health ecosystem, pharmacies already play a guiding role today and thus contribute to better cooperation among all participants in the health ecosystem, such as doctor's offices, hospitals, and care facilities (Fitte & Teuteberg, 2019; Frick & Schäfer, 2020). Pharmacies can, for example, take over the initial consultation for certain indications and thus contribute to a triage from which overloaded doctor's offices can benefit in terms of time and the health system can benefit financially. This also results in improved, interprofessional cooperation within the health sector, which often has a positive effect on therapy adherence, patient satisfaction, costs, and medication therapy safety (Fitte & Teuteberg, 2019). The contribution of pharmacies to the ecosystem is of particular importance for the latter. Unlike online pharmacies, local pharmacies maintain a better overview of their customers' overall medication, so that unwanted drug events such as drug interactions can be avoided, especially in the case of multimorbidity in older people (Hommel, 2018). To enable improved cooperation within a health ecosystem, a high degree of interdisciplinarity is required. Representatives of the various professions learn from each other in order to be able to adopt the perspectives of others and thus create a good basis for exchange with each other (Hommel, 2018).

8.1.2   Methodological Approach for the Survey of Experts

In April 2021, six semi-structured, guideline-based expert interviews were conducted with managers of pharmacies and drugstores from the distribution network of Dr. Bähler Dropa AG. The advantage of semi-structured expert interviews lies in the combination of a roughly predetermined structure with the possibility of asking spontaneous questions about unexpected new aspects and ambiguities (Meuser & Nagel, 2009). The developed guideline included questions about the professional situation of the interviewees, the service offerings of pharmacies, best practices (Bretschneider, 2004) in customer consulting, and collaboration within the health ecosystem. The thematic blocks resulted from the findings on the role of pharmacies in the health ecosystem from the four previous sub-studies of the present research project and the above-presented results of the literature search. With the choice, the focus of the interviews was placed on the promising future potentials of customer consulting and synergy development through cooperation in the ecosystem. The aim of the interviews was to identify proven best practices from the daily work of the interviewees for these areas and thus ensure a high practical relevance for the derivation of recommendations for action. An overview of the interviewed persons is provided in Table 8.1.

The 30-40 minute conversations were conducted via Zoom, recorded, and subsequently transcribed and coded in MAXQDA for evaluation purposes. The coding process utilized both deductive categories derived from the guidelines and inductive categories drawn from the material itself (Mayring, 2015). To ensure the reliability of these categories, the data was coded separately and independently by two researchers (Rädiker & Kuckartz, 2019). In the subsequent interpretation, the identified categories were condensed by the researchers into three thematic fields in an iterative process, within which

Table 8.1 Overview of the conducted expert interviews

	Interview 1	Interview 2	Interview 3	Interview 4	Interview 5	Interview 6
Place of Activity	Pharmacy and University	Pharmacy	Drugstore	Pharmacy	Pharmacy	Drugstore
Practical Experience	12 Years	20 Years	30 Years	12 Years	5 Years	35 Years
Gender	Male	Female	Female	Male	Male	Male

concrete recommendations for action were developed at the macro, meso, and micro levels of the health ecosystem.

8.2   Practical Experiences from Swiss Pharmacies and Drugstores

8.2.1   The Current Range of Services Offered by Pharmacies

The interviews revealed that the dispensing of medication remains the main reason why customers visit pharmacies today. However, there are a multitude of consultation services that are already being offered and used, such as emergency aid (Interview 1 and 5), travel medicine including vaccinations (Interview 1, 2, 4 and 5), and advice on specific topics such as skin problems or targeted advice for mothers (Interview 2 and 3). Many locations specialize in a particular area and communicate this to their customers. All interviewees reported successful service offerings in the field of natural medicine, such as spagyric medicine (Interview 1, 2 and 5) and hair mineral analysis (Interview 4).

According to four of the respondents, interprofessional collaboration in the context of triage is playing an increasingly important role in the range of services offered (Interview 1, 2, 4 and 6). For certain indications, pharmacies or drugstores serve as the first point of contact for those affected and offer a short-term available, qualified initial assessment. All respondents attribute this to the low-threshold access to the pharmacy due to good opening hours and advice without prior appointment or scheduling, as well as the cost advantage compared to a visit to the doctor's office, as also stated by interviewee 5: *"Many come with a problem and want to be advised. And many do not necessarily want to go to the doctor, because it is difficult to get an appointment and because they do not want to wait one or two weeks and it is associated with additional costs"*. In addition, trust in the pharmacy or in an independent second opinion is appreciated (Interview 1 and 4). Interviewee 6 also expresses this as follows: *"Of course, trust is important and that customers see us as trustworthy health advisors. This is already the case, otherwise we would not have any customers in the store"*. Also relevant for the choice of an initial consultation in the pharmacy is the high service orientation of the employees, for example through their focus on customer satisfaction (Interview 1 and 5).

8.2.2   Success Factors and Challenges for Customer Consultation in Pharmacies

According to all respondents, a high emphasis is placed on building a stable trusting relationship with customers in consultation services. The comparatively time-intensive consultation and the high willingness to solve problems play a role as success factors. If no one from the pharmacy can help, a solution is offered by referring to a doctor's office.

Interviewee 6 comments on this: *"They can also ask me questions that are not answered elsewhere. Even very simple questions, for which doctors no longer have time today. I spend a lot of time with people"*. For a consultation, appointments can be arranged, but usually this is not desired by customers, as the following statement from Interview 5 makes clear: *"...you don't have to make an appointment, you can just walk in and ask right away. Many consultations that we do are not chargeable"*.

Among the respondents, there is largely agreement that not all offers and competencies of pharmacy and drugstore employees are known to their customers. According to Interviewee 3, pharmacies primarily communicate their products, not their know-how. This leads to customers being surprised when, for example, vaccinations are also offered in pharmacies. Interviewee 2 comments on this as follows: *"The customers don't know everything that we offer (...). Even though it was advertised, many customers still don't know that we also vaccinate"*. Better communication of the services and competencies of pharmacies is also considered necessary towards doctors: *"The doctors don't know what the pharmacists do, there, communication also needs to be improved"* (Interview 1). The misjudgment by the various stakeholder groups about offers and competencies of pharmacies is attributed, among other things, to the lack of recognition within the health system (Interview 1, 4 and 6).

An additional challenge regarding the offer of consultation services for pharmacies is that a large part of the consultation services cannot be billed through health insurance. Customers expect the consultation in the pharmacy and drugstore to be free of charge: *"And at the moment they are used to not having to pay anything and it is a big step to be able to communicate to the customers why costs are now being added. That will be a big challenge"* (Interview 5). This coincides with shrinking margins for medications, which also increases the time pressure in the pharmacy. Accordingly, there is a strong desire to be able to bill consultation services in the pharmacy through health insurance (Interview 4).

Another challenge for the offer of consultation services in pharmacies is an inadequate infrastructure mentioned by the interviewees. Many locations are not designed for the provision of extensive services and in addition to the lack of separate consultation rooms (Interview 3), there is sometimes also a lack of qualified personnel to cover the entire opening hours of the pharmacy with consultation services (Interview 4).

To promote the awareness of the range of services beyond the dispensing of medication, additional offers are actively pointed out in the consultation. At many of the respondents' locations, traditional advertising in the form of posters, flyers and the website is also used, as well as special promotions and events: *"What was really great was when we showed the film 'The Pharmacist'. People talked about that for a long time"* (Interview 2). The recommendation by customers or "word-of-mouth" is also considered important (Interview 2 and 6). For this reason, a high level of satisfaction is highly valued.

8.2.3 Collaboration within the Health System

Within the healthcare system, pharmacies are already actively working with various partners. Foremost among these are doctor's offices in the immediate vicinity and specialized doctors, for example in dermatology. According to interviewee 1, collaboration between pharmacies and doctor's offices is promoted by the establishment of interprofessionalism already in the training of both disciplines. Accordingly, all respondents reported such collaborations and also rated them as beneficial: *"The exchange of knowledge is also good. For both sides it is helpful to be able to ask questions. The longer you know each other, the more likely you are to pick up the phone"* (Interview 4). In addition, the respondents appreciate an open exchange in local interprofessional quality circles as beneficial, as this facilitates, for example, referrals (Interview 2). This not only results in advantages for the respective cooperation partners, but also for the patients, e.g. saving time.

In addition to cooperation with doctor's offices, there are sometimes collaborations with the home care services Spitex (Interview 4 and 5) or with (senior) nursing homes (Interview 1 and 3). Cooperation with naturopathic practices was reported exclusively by the two managers of the drugstores in the interviews of the present study (Interview 3 and 6). The various collaborations are initiated equally by the pharmacies and drugstores as well as the respective cooperation partners.

In the context of the present research project and the focus on sustainable lifestyle change, explicit questions were asked about collaborations with nutritional counseling or providers of services to promote exercise. However, there have been no experiences in the sample examined, although some respondents consider cooperation with a nutritional counseling service to be quite interesting.

A particularly positively emphasized cooperation exists between some pharmacies and a Swiss health insurance company in connection to the topic of triage. Since certain consulting services can be provided more cost-effectively by pharmacies, the so-called pharmacy model of that health insurance company has established itself as a successful model: *"There is a collaboration with them in triage for eleven very specific indications in patients who have chosen the pharmacy model, they then come to us and are advised here. … This way, the family doctor's offices can be alleviated"* (Interview 4). This collaboration between pharmacies, doctor's offices and the health insurance company is a good example of the "task-shift" presented in Sect. 3.4, i.e. the transfer of tasks, with which expensive medical services are transferred to professions that work more cost-effectively (Schmelzer et al., 2020).

8.3 Conclusion

Today, pharmacies and drugstores in Switzerland play an important role within the healthcare system due to their nationwide, low-threshold access and high consulting competence. This could also be realized for the pursuit of a sustainable lifestyle change, as this often requires individual counseling, which could also be taken over by pharmacies or drugstores. In this context, the interviews conducted clarify development potentials especially in two areas: Firstly, there is a need for better communication of the offer and the competences of pharmacies and drugstores to strengthen their positions within the healthcare system. Particularly worth mentioning here are consulting services, for which, however, there are hardly any remuneration models so far. Secondly, by expanding the cooperation of the actors within the health ecosystem, synergies can be used more effectively. This is likely to result in advantages for all acting participants—the state, the health service providers and especially the customers.

References

Amazon Care. (n. d.). https://amazon.care/. Accessed 2. Dec. 2021.

Bretschneider, S. (2004). "Best practices" research: A methodological guide for the perplexed. *Journal of Public Administration Research and Theory, 15*(2), 307–323. https://doi.org/10.1093/jopart/mui017.

Fitte, C., & Teuteberg, F. (2019). Ein Rezept für die Apotheke 2.0: Wie Informations- und Kommunikationstechnologie die intersektorale Zusammenarbeit in der Gesundheitsversorgung stärken kann. *HMD Praxis der Wirtschaftsinformatik, 56*(1), 223–240. https://doi.org/10.1365/s40702-018-00485-3.

Frick, K., Bosshart, D., & Breit, S. (2020). *Next Health—Einfacher durch das Ökosystem der Gesundheit (GDI Trendreport)*. GDI Gottlieb Duttweiler Institute.

Frick, K., & Schäfer, C. (2020). *Apotheke 2030—Neue Modelle für ein Traditionsgeschäft (GDI Trendreport)*. GDI Gottlieb Duttweiler Institute.

Gerste, R. D. (2007). Retail Health Clinics: Medizin aus dem Supermarkt. *Deutsches Ärzteblatt, 104*(40), 2711–2712.

Hommel, T. (2018, March 10). Interdisziplinär gegen Risiken der Polypharmazie. *AerzteZeitung.de.* https://www.aerztezeitung.de/Kooperationen/Interdisziplinaer-gegen-Risiken-der-Polypharmazie-230300.html.

Leimeister, J. M. (2020). *Dienstleistungsengineering und -management: Data-driven service innovation* (2. ed.). Springer Gabler. https://doi.org/10.1007/978-3-662-59858-0.

Liat, Fishman Lea, Brühwiler David, Schwappach (2018). Medikationssicherheit: Wo steht die Schweiz?. Medication safety in Switzerland: Where are we today?. Bundesgesundheitsblatt—Gesundheitsforschung—Gesundheitsschutz 61(9) 1152–1158. https://doi.org/10.1007/s00103-018-2794-z

Martin, A., Brummond, P., Vlasimsky, T., Steffenhagen, A., Langley, J., Glowczewski, J., Boyd, A., Engels, M., Hermann, S., & Skaff, A. (2018). The evolving frontier of digital health: Opportunities for pharmacists on the horizon. *Hospital Pharmacy, 53*(1), 7–11. https://doi.org/10.1177/0018578717738221.

Mayring, P. (2015). *Qualitative Inhaltsanalyse: Grundlagen und Techniken* (12. ed.). Beltz.

Meuser, M., & Nagel, U. (2009). Das Experteninterview—Konzeptionelle Grundlagen und methodische Anlage. In S. Pickel, G. Pickel, H.-J. Lauth, & D. Jahn (Eds.), *Methoden der vergleichenden Politik- und Sozialwissenschaft: Neue Entwicklungen und Anwendungen* (pp. 465–479). VS Verlag. https://doi.org/10.1007/978-3-531-91826-6_23.

Pfeifer, J. (2014). German community pharmacists. *Nomos.* https://doi.org/10.5771/9783845255620.

pharmaSuisse (2020). Fakten und Zahlen Schweizer Apotheken. https://www.pharmasuisse.org/data/docs/de/19076/Fakten-und-Zahlen-2020.pdf

Rädiker, S., & Kuckartz, U. (2019). Intercoder-Übereinstimmung analysieren. In S. Rädiker & U. Kuckartz (Eds.), *Analyse qualitativer Daten mit MAXQDA* (pp. 287–303). Springer Fachmedien. https://doi.org/10.1007/978-3-658-22095-2_19.

Schmelzer, S., Hollenstein, E., Stahl, J., Wirz, M., Huber, M., Nast, I., & Liberatore, F. (2020). *Task Shifting in der inter-professionellen Zusammenarbeit*. ZHAW Zürcher Hochschule für Angewandte Wissenschaften. https://doi.org/10.21256/zhaw-20950.

Vargo, S. L., & Lusch, R. F. (2016). Institutions and axioms: An extension and update of service-dominant logic. *Journal of the Academy of Marketing Science, 44*(1), 5–23. https://doi.org/10.1007/s11747-015-0456-3.

Part III
Recommendations and Toolbox

Conclusion

9

Contents

Abstract

A variety of behavior change techniques support people with diabetes and obesity to change their lifestyle. Based on meta-analyses, measures are proposed which, from the perspective of those affected, are highly effective for a sustainable lifestyle change. In order to maintain a healthy lifestyle, measures that promote the autonomy of those affected prove to be promising. The challenge of sticking with it in the maintenance phase can be described in the form of a consumer journey. This phase is understood as an iterative process. If the maintenance of a healthy lifestyle is successful, those affected have a high degree of self-management, which is increasingly supported by technical aids that function as an "extended self". The design of the healthcare ecosystem also makes a relevant contribution to success. There is potential for optimization in areas such as interprofessionalism.

healthy lifestyle, this research project persued an interdisciplinary approach with various partner companies. The focus was on the so-called maintenance phase, that is, the phase of a change process in which the aim is to establish a new behavioural pattern – in this case a healthy lifestyle – in a sustainable way. Since old behavior patterns still represent a temptation in the maintenance phase, relapses (e.g., binge eating or skipping exercise sessions) are possible. In this maintanance stage people are faced with the challenge of overcoming obstacles, dealing with failures, and resisting temptations. In science and practice there are gaps in knowledge regarding the "sticking to" a healthy lifestyle, which this publication attempts to close. The interdisciplinary approach is reflected in the fact that the topic was examined from various disciplines and in this way motivational psychological approaches were combined with those of service management, in particular Transformative Service Research (TSR) and health economics. The collaboration of various scientific disciplines also involved a mix of quantitative and qualitative approaches.

The key findings are summarized in the following chapters and show how a healthy lifestyle can be successfully maintained.

9.1   Effective Measures for a Sustainable Lifestyle Change

This subchapter answers the following research question:

Which measures successfully support those affected in a sustainable lifestyle change?

A measure refers to the specific design and implementation of behavior change techniques (Behavior change techniques: BCTs). Since a variety of measures can be considered for a sustainable lifestyle change, the research question is answered by focusing on the underlying behavior change techniques. This approach allows for a systematic identification of effective behavior change techniques, from which appropriate measures can then be derived.

Table 9.1 lists the behavior change techniques which, according to meta-analyses (see Chap. 2), successfully support people with obesity or diabetes in lifestyle changes in the areas of exercise and nutrition. For a behavior change technique to be effective, it should be accepted and used by those affected. Because only the actual usage leads to a demonstrable effect of the measures (Hankonen et al., 2015). Table 9.1 therefore also shows which measures—based on the corresponding behavior change techniques—are particularly popular with those affected (see Chapts. 4 and 5).

Table 9.1 Catalogue of measures for effective behavior change techniques

Behavior change technique	Description	Area of behavior change	Popular with those affected
Behavioral goals (1.1)	Goal that describes a behavior	Physical Activity, Nutrition	YES
Problem solving (1.2)	Analyze behavior and develop strategies to overcome obstacles in pursuing goals	Nutrition	
Outcome goals (1.3)	Goal that describes an outcome	Physical Activity, Nutrition	YES
Action Planning (1.4)	Detailed planning of behavior	Physical Activity, Nutrition	YES
Feedback on Behavior (2.2)	Purely informative feedback on behaviors	Nutrition	YES
Self-Monitoring of Behavior (2.3)	Behavior is recorded by the person themselves	Physical Activity, Nutrition	YES
Feedback on Results (2.7)	Feedback on the results of behavior changes	Physical Activity, Nutrition	YES
Unspecific Social Support (3.1)	Arrange social support or provide information about it	Nutrition	YES
Instruction for Performing a Behavior (4.1)	Conveying the knowledge and skills to perform a behavior	Physical Activity, Nutrition	
Demonstration of Behavior (6.1)	Show desired behavior using an example	Physical Activity, Nutrition	
Social Comparison (6.2)	Practice behaviors in a safe framework	Nutrition	
Reduce Cue Signals (7.3)	Gradually reduce the stimulus that triggers the *desired* behavior	Nutrition	
Practice and Repeat Behavior (8.1)	Practice behaviors in a safe framework	Physical Activity, Nutrition	YES
Graded Tasks (8.7)	Start with simple tasks and gradually make them more difficult	Physical Activity, Nutrition	
Helpful Objects in the Environment (12.5)	Place an object that facilitates desired behavior in the environment	Physical Activity, Nutrition	

[Numbers in brackets refer to the numbering according to Michie et al. (2013)]

9.2   The Role of Motivation Orientation for Sustainable Lifestyle Change

The following research question is answered in this subchapter:

What role does motivation and motivation orientation play in maintaining a healthy lifestyle?

The motivation of those affected is the central element in changing and maintaining a healthy lifestyle. Because only the actual application of behavior change techniques leads to an effect of the measures (Hankonen et al., 2015). The application is based on the motivation of those affected themselves. The motivation can be either intrinsic, i.e., it is based on the joy or personal benefit of the action itself or the alignment with personal values. It can also be extrinsic in nature, i.e., it develops from outside through reward, pressure, or feelings of guilt (Hagger et al., 2020). It is important that those affected are intrinsically motivated to maintain a healthy lifestyle, as there is a correlation between intrinsic motivation orientation and successful behavior changes in the health sector (Ng et al., 2012; Sheeran et al., 2016).

With regard to the motivation orientation of the measures, it can be stated that these should be aimed at intrinsic motivation. This is achieved when measures optimally support the autonomy of those affected. The quantitative survey of those affected showed that measures that can be independently designed by those affected are more popular than measures that require support from external parties (e.g., professionals or personal environment) (see Chap. 5). Therefore, when designing measures, care should be taken to develop functions that individuals can use independently.

9.3   The Consumer Journey and the Customer Journeys in the Maintenance Phase

This subchapter answers the following research question:

What does the maintenance phase look like and what Customer Journey do those affected go through?

The research project revealed that the maintenance phase can be represented as a superordinate Consumer Journey with the goal of "maintaining a healthy lifestyle". The Consumer Journey has a overarching objective and includes several subordinate Customer Journeys. The Consumer Journey can be divided into three phases: At the beginning, there is always the objective, which includes not only the definition of a goal, but also the planning of activities to achieve this goal. In the second phase, the activities are implemented to achieve the desired goal. The third and final phase includes the review of goal achievement. Here, various variants could be identified based on the in-depth interviews. A fixed component of this phase is the "review of progress". However, the activities "receiving feedback" and "reward" are optional in the Consumer Journey. All study participants related this superordinate Consumer Journey to the two areas of exercise and nutrition in the interviews. This leads to the assumption that there are two Customer Journeys, which relate to physical activities and nutrition activities respectively, and that pursuing both Customer Journeys contributes to achieving the overarching objective of "maintaining a healthy lifestyle".

An important insight was gained with regard to the process character of the Customer Journey. The superordinate Consumer Journey and also the subordinate Customer Journeys are iterative processes. Those affected go through a process of behavior change again and again, which on a smaller scale is similar to the entire process of behavior change (cf. Sect. 2.1). The iterative character has two implications that are relevant for the assistence and support of those affected: 1) A sustainably healthy lifestyle will not happen by itself over time. Rather, those affected must constantly set themselves new goals in terms of exercise and nutrition in order to maintain the healthy lifestyle. This requires a high degree of motivation and discipline. 2) A sustainably healthy lifestyle can only be achieved if the goals relating to both nutrition and exercise are regularly achieved. Focusing on just one Customer Journey, i.e. either nutrition or exercise, is not promising.

Another open question was how positive emotions and motivation can be promoted during the maintenance phase. The study showed that a successful implementation of an activity (e.g. exercising, eating a healthy diet) is rated very positively by the 20 respondents. On a scale from 1 (very bad) to 5 (very good), this step in the Customer Journey achieved an average value of 4.5 (cf. Fig. 9.1). It should therefore be communicated more strongly to those affected that activities such as "exercising" or "eating a healthy diet" create a positive mood. It was also shown that the activities "receiving feedback" and "receiving reward" are associated with strong positive emotions. Eating a healthy and calorie-reduced dish or visiting a hip-hop course at the gym and exercising is rated as positively as receiving a reward. Although the two activities "receiving feedback" and "receiving reward" do not form an integral part of the Consumer Journey for all those affected. But especially when those affected are experiencing a low level of motivation, actively demanding feedback or a reward can be a strategy to bring oneself back into

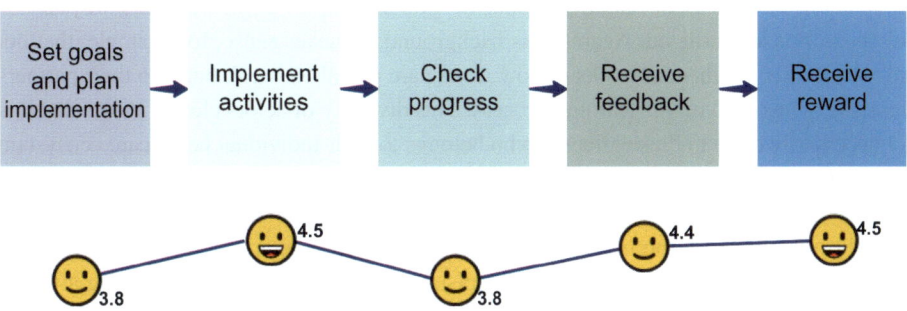

Fig. 9.1 Emotion curve during the Consumer Journey

a positive emotional state. Different forms of feedback and rewards have proven to be helpful: Feedback can take the form of recognition (for example, family members share their joy with those affected when they have achieved a goal in the field of physical exercise), but also in the form of comfort or assistance. In this case, for example, a conversation with a doctor or a nutritionist proves to be helpful. When it came to rewards bothmaterial forms (e.g. buying a new piece of clothing) and immaterial forms (e.g. recognition from friends) were mentioned.

9.4 The Healthcare Ecosystem: The Role of Those Affected and Their Partners in Maintaining a Healthy Lifestyle

This subchapter answers the following research question:

What role do those affected themselves and the other players in the healthcare ecosystem play in a long-term lifestyle change?

During their consumer journey "Maintaining a Healthy Lifestyle", affected individuals interact with various actors in the healthcare ecosystem. The healthcare ecosystem is a Service Business System: Various actors provide individual service parts, which together then result in a value-adding service. The common goal is to support those affected in pursuing a healthy lifestyle. In the healthcare ecosystem, the government assumes the role of the orchestrator, significantly determining the activities and resources of the other participants by shaping the healthcare system. The catalogue of basic insurance benefits offered by the health insurance providers is prescribed by the law. In the area of supplementary insurance, health insurance companies have more leeway, for example in the financial support of certain types of sports. They also act indirectly as orchestrators in this area. The premium system is more curative than preventive, thereby steering the behavior of those who use services. Service providers are doctors, nutritionists, physiotherapists and pharmacies. Complementary service providers (Service Contributors) include fitness studios and clubs, but also increasingly private companies, which often offer app-based support services for a healthy lifestyle. The social environment of those affected (Service Users), i.e. family members and friends, are important participants in the healthcare ecosystem. Their potential to act as Service Contributors and thus take an active part in the maintenance phase is not yet sufficiently utilized. Against this background, it makes sense, for example, that not only those affected themselves learn how to prepare a healthy meal, but also their partners are actively involved in this learning process. This diversity of actors clearly shows that it is not necessarily clear to those affected who belongs to their individual healthcare ecosystem and what roles the various actors can assume in interaction with them or with each other.

Which ecosystem actors are used by those affected individuals (Service Users) is strongly influenced by the orchestrators, but is ultimately determined very individually. For example, it is evident that physiotherapists play an important role for some affected people, while for others these providers of the healthcare ecosystem are not relevant. From the results of sub-study 2 (see Sect. 4.3.3) and the quantitative impact study (see

Sect. 5.4), it can be concluded that the collaboration of the various service providers is considered helpful by those affected and that the current degree of interprofessionalism clearly offers room for improvement. A higher degree of interprofessionalism would lead to a win-win situation: Not only do those affected appreciate being jointly cared for by a doctor and a nutritionist and benefiting from their specialist knowledge. The healthcare system and thus society can also benefit from lower costs, as services of nutritionists are cheaper than those of doctors. The results of the qualitative impact study (see Chap. 7) and the study on pharmacies (see Chap. 8) point in the same direction. The potential of pharmacies and drugstores to support those affected to maintain a healthy lifestyle is still significantly underutilized. More intensive collaboration between doctors and pharmacies and drugstores brings a higher service quality for affected people (fast, direct advice without an appointment) and helps to reduce bottlenecks in medical care.

Self-management plays an important role in maintaining a healthy lifestyle. This finding is clearly supported by the quantitative impact study (see Chap. 5). Therefore, it is important that those affected are aware of the significance of their own actions. In the step "Implementing Activities" in the consumer journey and also in dealing with challenges self-management is particulary important. However, this does not mean that the other actors in the healthcare ecosystem lose importance. On the contrary: doctors, family and friends play a crucial role in maintaining a healthy lifestyle and those affected desire more social support from these actors. The quantitative impact study (see Chap. 5) also showed that the healthcare ecosystem becomes more important the older those affected are. This was expressed by a significant difference in survey results from people aged up to 63 years and the older comparison group (64 to 82 years). Support from actors in the healthcare ecosystem such as medical professionals, people in the same household, and health insurance companies are considered more valuable by older people in comparison.

Social support can be provided in different ways: emotional, instrumental, and informational (House, 1981). According to the results of the qualitative impact study (see Chap. 7), those affected desire more emotional support from both doctors and their private environment, for example, to comfort them when they complain about how difficult it is to eat a healthy diet or when they fall back into unhealthy eating habits. More instrumental support, to carry out a specific action and thus help those affected, is primarily expected from their circle of friends. For instance, it is considered helpful if the hosts serve a calorie-reduced meal at a dinner invitation, without those affected having to explain or justify themselves. In terms of informational support (e.g., giving tips on how to make vegetables tasty), those affected see less need for themselves, but rather for their family members. This can be attributed to the fact that those affected have already built up knowledge about healthy eating and sufficient exercise during the maintenance phase. The potential of the private environment (family and circle of friends) should therefore be used more intensively. For example, it may be useful for not only those affected to receive important information during nutritional counseling, but also for their partners to be involved.

Even if, according to the quantitative impact study (see Chap. 5), the use of technical aids decreases with the increasing age of those affected, there is nevertheless a clear trend towards a growing importance of these aids for maintaining a healthy lifestyle. Technical aids can increase the autonomy of those affected and also enable networking between the players in the healthcare ecosystem. These aids are often app-based and offered by service contributors. They support those affected in their self-management and perform functions that were previously often performed by doctors. For example, certain checks (e.g., blood sugar or blood pressure checks) can be carried out by those affected themselves. Therefore, technical aids are referred to as "Extended Self". Technical aids are used in particular for goal setting and monitoring, i.e., checking progress. Those affected also increasingly rely on the use of digital tools in communication with service providers. In this respect, a development of the healthcare ecosystem towards a digital healthcare ecosystem (Digital Business Ecosystem, see Sect. 3.3) would be desirable. The use of digital tools should be a supplement, as those affected emphasize that face-to-face contact is still very important. Digital Business Ecosystems offer the advantage that the use of information and communication technologies facilitates networking of ecosystem actors. In addition, those affected have access to their own health data at any time, which supports them in maintaining a healthy lifestyle. The company Uplyfe, one of the business partner in the research project, is taking this path: those affected get an overview of their own data, which supports their self-management. They can also connect with a nutritionist via chat in emergency situations and get advice. Uplyfe has entered into cooperations with various other actors in the healthcare ecosystem (e.g., health insurance companies, doctor networks), which ultimately leads to a higher service quality for those affected, as they experience effective and efficient support in the maintenance phase.

9.5   Conclusion

The results of the interdisciplinary research project show that "sticking to" a healthy lifestyle is an iterative process and therefore cannot be regarded as a final phase. How successfull "sticking to it" is, depends on the motivation of those affected and the organisation of support measures. Measures have been identified that are particularly effective for this phase. The self-management of those affected plays an important role for sustainable lifestyle change. Therefore, measures and support from ecosystem partners should be aimed at increasing the autonomy of those affected. Finally, it was shown that there is considerable potential in the design of the healthcare ecosystem. By increasing interprofessionalism, it would be possible to increase value for those affected through high service quality as well as cost savings that benefit society.

References

Hagger, M. S., Hankonen, N. E., & Ryan, R. M. (2020). Changing behavior using self-determination theory. *The handbook of behavior change* (pp. 104–119). Cambridge University Press. https://doi.org/10.1017/9781108677318.008.

Hankonen, N., Sutton, S., Prevost, A. T., Simmons, R. K., Griffin, S. J., Kinmonth, A. L., & Hardeman, W. (2015). Which behavior change techniques are associated with changes in physical activity, diet and body mass index in people with recently diagnosed diabetes? *Annals of Behavioral Medicine: A Publication of the Society of Behavioral Medicine, 49*(1), 7–17. https://doi.org/10.1007/s12160-014-9624-9.

House, J. S. (1981). *Work stress and social support.* Addison-Wesley Pub. Co.

Michie, S., Richardson, M., Johnston, M., Abraham, C., Francis, J., Hardeman, W., Eccles, M. P., Cane, J., & Wood, C. E. (2013). The behavior change technique taxonomy (v1) of 93 hierarchically clustered techniques: Building an international consensus for the reporting of behavior change interventions. *Annals of Behavioral Medicine, 46*(1), 81–95. https://doi.org/10.1007/s12160-013-9486-6.

Ng, J. Y. Y., Ntoumanis, N., Thøgersen-Ntoumani, C., Deci, E. L., Ryan, R. M., Duda, J. L., & Williams, G. C. (2012). Self-determination theory applied to health contexts: A meta-analysis. *Perspectives on Psychological Science, 7*(4), 325–340. https://doi.org/10.1177/1745691612447309.

Sheeran, P., Maki, A., Montanaro, E., Avishai-Yitshak, A., Bryan, A., Klein, W. M. P., Miles, E., & Rothman, A. J. (2016). The impact of changing attitudes, norms, and self-efficacy on health-related intentions and behavior: A meta-analysis. *Health Psychology: Official Journal of the Division of Health Psychology, American Psychological Association, 35*(11), 1178–1188. https://doi.org/10.1037/hea0000387.

Toolbox for Maintaining a Healthy Lifestyle

10

Contents

Abstract

The toolbox is a compilation of practical tools to support a sustainable lifestyle change. It is aimed at health service providers such as doctors, health coaches, nutritionists, and pharmacists. They can use tools from the toolbox to help individuals maintaining a healthy lifestyle. The various tools compiled in the toolbox are based on findings from existing literature as well as insights gathered during the interdisciplinary research project.

Maintaining a healthy lifestyle is a challenge for those affected with health issues. Diet and exercise programs do indeed support the transition to a healthy lifestyle, but once the enthusiasm over the lost kilos and gained muscles has faded, many fall back into old patterns. If this happens repeatedly, it is referred to as the yo-yo effect. The challenges of everyday life—such as balancing work and family—and the power of habit are possible explanations for the relapse into an unhealthy lifestyle: Nutrition becomes less conscious again, exercise is reduced, and often the initial weight is quickly regained or, in the worst case, even exceeded. What can and should the various actors in the health care ecosystem do to best support those affected in maintaining a healthy lifestyle?

The toolbox presented here offers professionals in the health system assistance for optimal support of those affected in the phase of maintaining the changed lifestyle. The toolbox consists of eight elements that can be used during the consultation and support of the target audience in the maintenance stage of a healthy lifestyle:

- Tool 1—Customer Journey: What steps do those affected go through when they want to maintain a healthy lifestyle, and what should be considered in their design?
- Tool 2—Map of the Health Care Ecosystem: Who are the relevant actors in the health care ecosystem and what role do they and those affected play in maintaining a healthy lifestyle?
- Tool 3—Collaboration and Interprofessionalism in the Health Care Ecosystem: What possibilities for collaboration among the various actors in the health care ecosystem exist and how do they support those affected through this collaboration?
- Tool 4—Effective and Practical Behavior Change Techniques: Which behavior change techniques are particularly effective with regards to nutrition and exercise and are also acceptedby the target audience?
- Tool 5—Guide to Autonomy-Oriented Design of Measures: How can measures be designed to optimally support the autonomy of those affected?
- Tool 6—Individual Goal Setting: How can meaningful and individually suitable goals be set?
- Tool 7—Short Questionnaire on the Acceptance of Measures and Motivation Orientation: How can the acceptance of individual measures be captured and accounted for? How can it be checked to what extent the lifestyle change is based on intrinsic or extrinsic motivation?
- Tool 8—Guide to Defining Appropriate Rewards: What are the options for optimal rewards?

The initial situation for the support and guidance of people who want to shape their lifestyle sustainably healthy is very different for the various actors in the health care ecosystem. Content, intensity, and duration vary and are situation-specific as well as person-dependent. Thus, the initial situation for support in a long-term relationship between those affected and their doctors is easier than in a situation where rather spontaneous tips are given by employees in the gym. Moreover, the transition to a sustainable, healthy lifestyle is different for each person and the consultation processes are correspondingly diverse. Therefore, the toolbox presented here provides a selection of tools that can be personalised. For the various actors in the health care ecosystem, it is important to find out which of the tools are most promising to use for which consultation with which person.

10.1   Tool 1: Customer Journey

As a basis for consultation on maintaining a healthy lifestyle, those affected should be made aware of the peculiarities of the Customer Journey of the maintenance stage. It is recommended to illuminate the phases of the Customer Journey step by step with them. The following aspects should be considered:

- In order to pursue a healthy lifestyle sustainably, it is important that those affected change their diet *and* exercise sufficiently. This has implications for all phases of the Customer Journey (see below). Focusing solely on one of the two areas, for example by greatly increasing physical activities, but without adjusting a possibly unhealthy diet, does not lead to succesful goal achievement.
- A sustainably healthy lifestyle is not getting established automatically. Those affected should be made aware of how important it is that they continually set new goals in terms of nutrition and exercise and regularly check their achievement.

To make the maintenance stage as efficient as possible for those affected, it is recommended to illuminate the individual steps using Tool 1 "Customer Journey". Fig. 10.1 provides information about the individual steps as well as the connection to other tools and shows what needs to be considered.

10.2   Tools for the Health Care Ecosystem

Tools 2 and 3 were developed to clarify the roles and offers of the various actors within the health care ecosystem. The tools show where there is potential from the perspective of interprofessionalism to successfully support those affected in the maintenance stage.

The main identified actors in the health care ecosystem are represented in the ecosystem map (see Fig. 10.2). Two central findings were obtained from the studies:

- Those affected usually name one person as the most important support for their lifestyle change. This is often their (family) doctor, a nutrition counselor, or a person from their social environment.
- People from the social environment play a very important role when it comes to the sustainable success of a lifestyle change. These people can be more strongly involved in the support of those affected: They have a direct positive motivational influence

Activities of the customer journey	What needs to be considered?	Other relevant tools
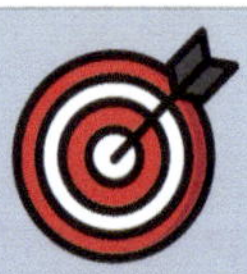 **Set goals and plan implementation**	A combination of nutrition and exercise goals should be formulated in each case. It is important to set both long-term goals and intermediate goals so that those affected do not feel overwhelmed. Ideally, the goals should be written down and a target date should be noted for each goal.	2 3 4 5
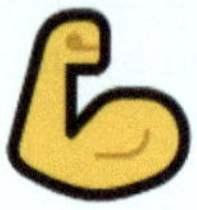 **Implement activities**	The realization of the activities triggers feelings of happiness! Those affected should be aware of this so that they can motivate themselves to be active more easily.	2 3 4 5
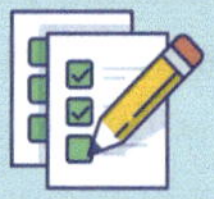 **Check progress**	Checking your progress (including intermediate goals) helps you to see where you stand. Technical aids (e.g. pedometers on your cell phone) can help with this. Reaching your goal has a motivating effect. If you miss your target, you can consider correcting it.	5 6 7
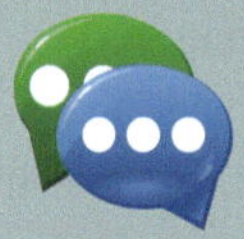 **Receive feedback**	Looking at the pedometer or the scales is one form of feedback. However, it can be particularly helpful in difficult moments to actively seek feedback, e.g. from your partner when you have managed to walk 4,000 steps in one go.	5 7
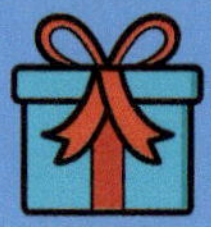 **Receive reward**	Rewards can be tangible or intangible (see Tool 8). Especially in challenging situations, it can help if you actively "demand" a reward: be it in the form of rewarding yourself or actively seeking feedback in the form of recognition or support from a trusted person.	8

Fig. 10.1 Phases of the Customer Journey and relevant tools

on the person's decisions regarding their lifestyle and can also be integrated into the system of reward and feedback. Friends thus relieve professional (and therefore fee-based) health service providers by successfully "partially" substituting their tasks due to their closer proximity to the person. This leads to an overall relief of the healthcare system.

In order to advise those affected well and to build on previous measures and successes, it is recommended to ask at the first contact with affected individuals which other actors have already been involved in the lifestyle change or were. Based on this, further helpful

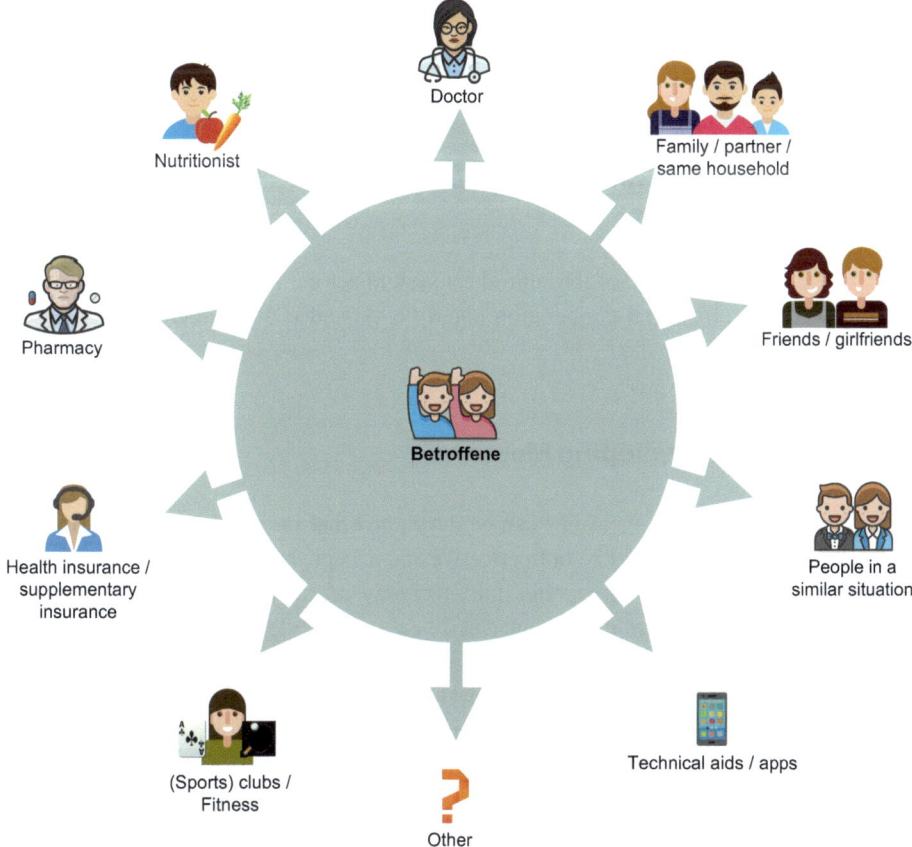

Fig. 10.2   Tool 2 Network of ecosystem actors to promote interprofessionalism

actors can be suggested and their potential role discussed (Tool 2). Tool 3 can also be
used to show the potential networking between all participants.

10.2.1 Tool 2: Health Care Ecosystem Map

The representation of the most relevant ecosystem actors in the form of a clear map
is intended to make affected individuals aware of the variety of possible actors. In
Fig. 10.2, the groups of people identified as central in the project are found. Of course,
other health professionals (e.g., specialists) may be important in individual cases. Here,
the focus is on the most important actors in the area of sustainable lifestyle change.
These include the doctor, nutrition counseling, pharmacy, health insurance, sports clubs
and fitness studios, family, partner, people of the same household, friends, and people

in a similar situation. Since technical aids are playing an increasingly important role in maintaining a healthy lifestyle and are offered by health service providers, they are also listed in the health care ecosystem map.

10.2.2 Tool 3: Collaboration and Interprofessionalism in the Health Care Ecosystem

Table 10.1 describes the role of the central ecosystem actors. In addition, it shows for all actors how interprofessional cooperation could be expanded and which actors are particularly suitable for this.

10.3   Tools for Developing Measures

Tools 4 to 8 illustrate how measures can be developed that promote sustainable lifestyle changes. The measures should be both effective and accepted and used by those affected. Only when measures can be integrated into everyday life and are used with enjoyment and commitment a long-term maintenance of a healthy lifestyle can emerge.

With Tool 4, effective and practical behavior change techniques are described, on the basis of which suitable measures can be developed in collaboration with those affected. A distinction is made between behavior change techniques for measures for physical activity and behavior change techniques for measures for nutrition.

Tool 5 proposes measures that promote autonomy in those affected. High autonomy supports the long-term maintenance of behavior changes.

Tool 6 provides guidance for individual goal setting. For long-term behavior changes, both goal setting at the beginning and regular monitoring and adjustment of goals and corresponding intermediate goals are important.

Tool 7 offers two short questionnaires for assessing the acceptance of a measure and the motivation orientation of those affected. The acceptance of a measure promotes its use, intrinsic motivation supports the long-term maintenance of behavior changes.

Tool 8 proposes possibilities for selecting suitable rewards. Rewards should be designed in such a way that they motivate those affected and at the same time promote their autonomy.

10.3.1 Tool 4: Effective and Practical Behavior Change Techniques

For a behavior change towards a healthy lifestyle, a coordinated set of activities for physical activity and nutrition is required, the so-called *intervention*. The intervention includes certain *behavior change techniques,* which represent "active ingredients" and

Table 10.1   Tool 3 Relevant actors in the health care ecosystem

Actor	Role in the health care ecosystem and opportunities for collaboration	Potential for collaboration
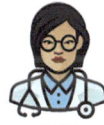 Doctor	(Family-) doctors play a very central role in the lifestyle change of many affected people and are often mentioned as the most important supporters in this process. This is due to the fact that they are usually the first contact for people with health problems and they often maintain long-term relationships with their patients. They generally enjoy a high reputation and take on an important interface function in the health system by ensuring the coordination of interprofessional treatment (for example with physiotherapy or nutritionist). At the same time, the use of services by doctors is associated with comparatively high costs for the health system as a whole and sometimes also for those affected themselves. Many successful examples can already be observed for cooperation within the health care ecosystem: inclusion of other providers of health services in the same practice (e.g. nutritionist), exchange in quality circles with their own or other professions, or close cooperation with pharmacies and drugstores. A successful example is the so-called pharmacy model for optimized triage regarding various diagnoses, for which recognition and cost coverage by the health insurance company is required.	Nutritionist Pharmacy Family / partner / same household Health insurance
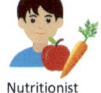 Nutritionist	Nutritional counseling was mentioned in the studies alongside the doctor as the most important support for the transition to a healthy lifestyle. Through the individual support of those affectedover a certain period of time, stable relationships of trust often develop. There are connections between nutritionistg and doctors, and there is also a relationship with health insurance companies through cost reimbursement. Here too, it is recommended to involve people from the social environment of those affected, as a common solution with family members or partner must usually be found in terms of eating. Since the combination of nutritional and exercise goals is of very high importance, expanding cooperation with exercise providers such as physiotherapists and fitness studios has high potential. The increasing importance of technical aids such as apps and consultations via chat is likely to have a strong impact on the work of nutritional counseling. Especially among younger target groups and among people with whom a personal relationship has already been established, a high acceptance of such offers can be expected.	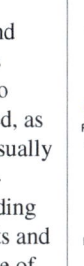

(continued)

Table 10.1 (continued)

Actor	Role in the health care ecosystem and opportunities for collaboration	Potential for collaboration
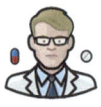 Pharmacy	According to the studies conducted, pharmacies so far play a subordinate role in advising on healthy lifestyle changes, although they have high potential in this area. Especially because of the low-threshold access to pharmacies, they could perform additional consulting services. Possible examples include recommendations for a healthy diet and more exercise, monitoring of health data through measurements in the pharmacy, or even the evaluation of data from health apps. Due to the low-threshold access to pharmacies, not only an expansion of services for those affected is offered, but especially the inclusion of people from the social environment of those affected. Seminars at the pharmacy on relevant topics (e.g. lowering cholesterol levels) are recommended, where people in similar situations could exchange ideas or where other family members and acquaintances could also come along to find out how they can support those affected in their lifestyle change. To enable better cooperation with other actors in the health care ecosystem, better recognition of pharmacies as part of the health care ecosystem and more adequate reimbursement of consulting services by health insurance companies is needed. The pharmacy model of certain health insurance companies serves as a successful example here. However, so far it only refers to selected diagnoses and not to preventive consulting services. Exactly there, however, there is enormous potential to improve the long-term health of the population and reduce health costs.	 Doctor Family / partner / same household Health insurance
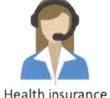 Health insurance	Health insurance companies also play a rather subordinate role in the health care ecosystem from the perspective of those affected. They are primarily perceived as pure payers and less as service providers who can support with additional offers. This applies not only to those affected, but also with regard to doctors, therapists, and private service providers such as fitness studios, for example. To strengthen the role of health insurance, additional offers such as health coaches are recommended, who can advise those affected on their options for changing their lifestyle or draw attention to promoted services. Health insurance companies should support and promote this form of prevention more strongly. The communication of such service offers needs to be expanded so that those affected can also perceive the new role that their health insurance can take on.	 Doctor Nutritional advice Pharmacy Technical aids / Apps (Sports) clubs / Fitness

(continued)

Table 10.1   (continued)

Actor	Role in the health care ecosystem and opportunities for collaboration	Potential for collaboration
 (Sports) clubs / Fitness	Compared to prescribed exercise programs such as physiotherapy, sports clubs and especially fitness studios offer low-threshold offers that have been very popular for many years. This is consistent with the findings from the studies conducted. The reasons mentioned include above all the possibility of combining exercise with social exchange. While some people appreciate the flexible access to fitness offers, it is helpful for others to establish a certain routine or (social) pressure through fixed weekly appointments. People from the social environment are also of great importance for the use of exercise offers in clubs and fitness studios. The potential of this role can be further exploited through targeted actions such as "Bring a friend", a "Family Day" or special discounts for joint training—not only by the service providers themselves, but possibly also by the supplementary insurances of the health insurance companies.	Friends Family / partner / same household Health insurance
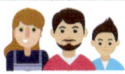 Family / partner / same household	The social environment of those affected plays a very important role in the transition to a healthy lifestyle. It can favor the change, but also hinder it. Accordingly, family, partners, and people living in the same household are on par with doctors or nutritionist in terms of their importance, even if their contributions to lifestyle change take a completely different form. Favorable effects include, for example, active participation in new behaviors such as regular walking or jogging and the joint renunciation of certain foods or the cooking and enjoyment of healthy meals. In contrast, the change can be made more difficult if the social environment does not take any consideration of the intended lifestyle change of the person concerned or even expresses itself negatively about it. Almost all actors in the health care ecosystem have the opportunity to involve people from the social environment of those affected in order to promote a healthy lifestyle. If information from professional providers is shared with them, they can adapt their behavior in such a way that they can support and motivate those affected. They can become aware of setbacks early on and support those affected in this situation in a targeted manner. Joint activities such as cooking courses or exercise offers (see sports clubs/fitness) are considered particularly conducive to the use of the potential of this group of people.	Doctor Nutritional advice Technical aids / Apps Pharmacy (Sports) clubs / Fitness

(continued)

Table 10.1 (continued)

Actor	Role in the health care ecosystem and opportunities for collaboration	Potential for collaboration
Friends People in a similar situation	Similar to family or partners, friends can also play a crucial role in maintaining a healthy lifestyle, for example, by making arrangements for joint beneficial behaviors such as exercise or healthy eating. However, unlike people living in the same household, the topic of nutrition plays a somewhat lesser role here, as shopping and food preparation are rarely done together. Friends play a particularly important role when it comes to, for example, signing up for a sports club together. In addition, they can take on a reinforcing, motivating function if they stay in contact with those affected via technical aids such as chat and social media, praise and encourage healthy behavior.	Technical aids / apps (Sports) clubs / Fitness
People in a similar situation	The importance of people in a similar situation was rated very differently by the respondents in the studies conducted. For some, this group of people plays no role, for others they are very important, as those affected feel better understood by them than by people from their social environment. Contact with people in a similar situation either comes about in self-help groups (e.g., Weight Watchers), at the gym, or through technical aids such as online forums and social media like Facebook groups. Improved cooperation with people in similar situations can be initiated by various professional actors such as doctor's offices, pharmacies, health insurance companies, and nutritional counseling. This could be realized through the organization of theme events or by referring to appropriate forums.	Technical aids / apps

Technical aids / apps	Under the collective term "technical aids", the respondents in the studies understood aids such as pedometers, scales, and especially various types of apps. These apps include those that offer entire health programs such as Uplyfe, apps for monitoring exercise such as pedometers or running apps, but also social media apps like Facebook and WhatsApp. Such apps are used during the maintenance stage primarily for the activities "setting goals" and "checking progress" (monitoring). Increasingly, communication with actors from the health care ecosystem is gaining importance, for example, the exchange of messages with the physiotherapist or nutritionist.
	Technical aids are established and popular in all age groups (with exceptions > 64 years). It can be assumed that the importance of technical aids will continue to increase. Therefore, it is advisable for professional actors in the health care ecosystem to already think about how they can combine their services with technical aids. An example of this is the offer from health insurance companies for additional insurance, linking rewards to the transmission of data from wearables or apps to steps taken. Within the social environment of those affected, technical aids are already being used, for example, by setting and tracking common goals via chat or by people in similar situations finding each other in online groups.
		Nutritional advice
		
		  Friends
		
		  Family / partner / same household
		
		  Health insurance
		
		  People in a similar situation

Table 10.1   (continued)

Actor	Role in the health care ecosystem and opportunities for collaboration	Potential for collaboration
? Other	In addition to the mentioned actors, other support possibilities are feasible, e.g., through specialist literature on a healthy lifestyle, cookbooks/recipes, pets (especially dogs and cats), coaching/psychotherapy, physiotherapy, diabetes counseling, or the gastronomy with offers and information on healthy dishes and ingredients.	

influence the processes of behavior change. The design and implementation of a behavior change technique represents the concrete *measure*.

Through a literature search, the effective behavior change techniques for the two areas of physical activity and nutrition were identified (see Chap. 2). These are listed below, described and illustrated with an example for a corresponding measure (see Table 10.2 and 10.3).

In the first study conducted as part of the research project (see Chap. 4), interviews with those affected were used to determine which behavior change techniques they frequently used and which are therefore relevant from their point of view. These techniques are marked with a yellow star in Tables 10.2 and 10.3.

Physical activity

The following behavior change techniques are effective according to meta-analyses for measures to promote physical activity. (see Table 10.2)

Nutrition

The following behavior change techniques are effective for promoting healthy nutrition according to meta-analyses. (see Table 10.3)

10.3.2 Tool 5: Guide to Autonomy-Oriented Design of Measures

Behavioral changes are more sustainable when they occur due to the individual's intrinsic motivation (Ng et al., 2012). Therefore, it is important to promote autonomy in those affected so that behavioral changes can be maintained independently. Measures should be designed to allow a high degree of autonomy. The following elements can be used to design measures in the various stages of lifestyle change and maintenance in an autonomy-oriented way (see Table 10.4).

Table 10.2 Effective behavior change techniques for physical activity interventions

Behavior change technique	Description	Exemplary measure
Behavioral goals (1.1) ⭐	Goal that describes a behavior	Run five kilometers three times a week
Outcome goals (1.3) ⭐	Goal that describes an outcome	Be able to run ten kilometers at a stretch in three months
Action planning (1.4) ⭐	Detailed planning of the behavior	Run every Monday morning from 8:00–8:45
Self-monitoring of behavior (2.3) ⭐	Behavior is recorded by the person themselves	Diary with physical activities
Feedback on outcomes (2.7) ⭐	Feedback on the outcomes of behavior changes	Fitness instructor gives feedback on muscle mass increase
Instruction on how to perform a behavior (4.1)	Conveying the knowledge and skills to perform a behavior	Fitness instructor shows simple fitness exercises for home use
Demonstration of behavior (6.1)	Show desired behavior using an example	Read a blog of a person affected to get inspiration on how to incorporate physical activity into everyday life
Behavioural practice / rehearsal (8.1)	Practice behaviors in a safe setting	Practice simple fitness exercises with fitness instructor
Graded tasks (8.7)	Start with simple tasks and gradually make them more difficult	Start with brisk walks, then small jogging rounds, until the person can run five kilometers
Adding objects to the environment (12.5)	Place an object that facilitates desired behavior in the environment	Set up a trampoline in the living room to take regular active breaks

Note. The numbering of the behavior change techniques refers to the classification according to Michie et al. (2013)

10.3.3   Tool 6: Individual Goal Setting

Setting goals for behavioral objectives, e.g., for physical activities, and outcome goals, e.g., for weight reduction, are effective and are also accepted by those affected (see Sect. 10.3.1). Thus, setting goals is an important element of behavior change, especially

Table 10.3 Effective behavior change techniques for measures in the field of nutrition

Behavior change technique	Description	Exemplary measure
Behavioral goals (1.1) ⭐	Goal that describes a behavior	Cook a healthy meal five times a week
Problem solving (1.2)	Analyze behavior and develop strategies to overcome obstacles in pursuing goals	Because the person is too tired to cook after work, they prepare the meals for the next week on Sunday
Outcome goals (1.3) ⭐	Goal that describes an outcome	Lose two kilos within a month
Action planning (1.4) ⭐	Detailed planning of behavior	Prepare meals on Sunday afternoon from 2:00–4:00
Feedback on behavior (2.2)	Purely informative feedback on behaviors	Feedback on healthy eating habits based on a questionnaire
Self-monitoring of behavior (2.3) ⭐	Behavior is recorded by the person themselves	Diary with the meals consumed daily
Feedback on the results (2.7) ⭐	Feedback on the results of behavior changes	Doctor gives feedback on the amount of weight loss
Instruction for performing a behavior (4.1) ⭐	Conveying the knowledge and skills to perform a behavior	Health app suggests healthy meals
Demonstration of behavior (6.1)	Show desired behavior using an example	Read a blog of a person affected to get inspiration for healthy meals
Social Comparison (6.2)	Encourage comparison with other people	Compare weight loss with other affected individuals
Behavioural Practice / rehearsal (8.1)	Practice behaviors in a safe framework	Attend a cooking course on fiber-rich vegetarian cuisine
Graded Tasks (8.7)	Start with simple tasks and gradually make them more difficult	Start with two healthy meals a week, then gradually increase until you reach five healthy meals
AddingObjects to the Environment (12.5)	Place an object that facilitates desired behavior in the environment	Keep a cookbook with healthy recipes within reach in the kitchen

Note. The numbering of the behavior change techniques refers to the classification according to Michie et al. (2013)

Table 10.4 Autonomy-Oriented Design of Measures

Area of Measures	Quality Criterion for Design of Interventions	Quality Criterion for Ecosystem Partners
Goal Setting	Long-term goals that can be achieved in various ways	Peer-level feedback
	Offer diverse options for goals	Performance-oriented communication
	Set pace yourself	Feedback for performance improvement
	Enable self-monitoring (e.g., with wearables)	General approach instead of control
	Allow room for action (e.g., Cheat-Day)	Offer examples from other users as ideas
Measures	Only hints on measures (Pull instead of Push)	Variety of possible goals
	Broad selection of measures	Performance measurement
	Selection of different channels	Independent determination of the ratio of internalization/externalization
	Choice regarding type of feedback and communication	High responsiveness
		Availability of facilities/service providers
		Empowerment
Ecosystem Partners	Professional communication at eye level	Digital channels
	Accessibility via various channels	Prompts on channels without obligation
		High usability of mobile devices/channels
		Accessibility in case of problems

in the preparation phase and the action stage. But even in the maintenance stage, it is important to constantly reviewing one's own goals and setting new goals if necessary. Therefore, intermediate goals are also very relevant. The goal setting can be flexible and be constantly adapted to changing circumstances and goal changes: A main goal can have several intermediate goals, and a main goal can later become an intermediate goal when a new main goal is set. However, it is important that the goals are reviewed and the progress is monitored. The monitoring can be done by an external person or through self-monitoring. It is also important that goals are always set for the two areas of physical activity and nutrition.

In Table 10.5, an exemplary guide for individual goal agreements with those affected is given.

Table 10.5   Guide for Individual Goal Setting

Area		Type of Goal	Example	Monitoring
		Outcome Goal (Main Goal)	After 3 months: 12 kg less	Weight measurement after 3 months
		Outcome Goal (Intermediate Goal)	Every 4 weeks: 4 kg less	Weight measurement every four weeks
	Additional Outcome Goals as Needed			
		Behavioral Goal (Main Goal)	No consumption of sugary drinks	Check with food diary
		Behavioral Goal (Intermediate Goal)	Max. 3 sugary drinks per week	Check with food diary
		Behavioral Goal (Main Goal)	2h physical activity (swimming, jogging etc.) per week	Check with activity diary
		Behavioral Goal (Intermediate Goal 1)	4 × 30 min everyday exercise per week	Check with activity diary
		Behavioral Goal (Intermediate Goal 2)	2 × 30 min everyday exercise + 2 × 30 min physical activity per week	Check with activity diary
	Additional Behavioral Goals as Needed			

10.3.4 Tool 7: Short Questionnaire on the Acceptance of Measures and Motivation Orientation

For a digital measure to be effective, it must be accepted and used by those affected.

To measure acceptance, the questions documented in the following table should be answered for each measure (see Table 10.6). The rule is: the higher the values, the more the measure is accepted. It makes sense to recommend to those affected only such measures that are also accepted.

Table 10.6   Short questionnaire on the acceptance of measures

Question	Category	Response Scale
I would enjoy using this measure	Acceptance	1 "Strongly disagree" to 5 "Strongly agree"
This measure could be easily integrated into my daily routine	Acceptance	1 "Strongly disagree" to 5 "Strongly agree"
This measure would be useful to me	Acceptance	1 "Strongly disagree" to 5 "Strongly agree"

Behavior changes are maintained in the long term when they occur due to intrinsic motivation (Ng et al., 2012). Intrinsic motivation involves an action being carried out due to enjoyment of the action itself, due to personal benefit, or due to alignment with personal values (Hagger et al., 2020). In contrast, behavior in the case of extrinsic motivation occurs due to reward, social pressure, or to avoid feelings of guilt.

Therefore, across all measures, the questions compiled in the table on motivation orientation should be answered (see Table 10.7). The intrinsic motivation orientation is more pronounced the higher the values of the responses on the response scale for intrinsic motivation and the lower the values on the response scale for extrinsic motivation.

If intrinsic motivation is low, or extrinsic motivation is high, further measures to promote intrinsic motivation should be considered.

10.3.5 Tool 8: Guide to Defining Appropriate Rewards

Rewards are important for successful lifestyle changes and maintenance. At the same time, those affected should be encouraged in their autonomy so that they can independently maintain behavioral changes. Therefore, it is also important to design the rewards in an autonomy-oriented way and to offer those affected a selection of different rewards (see Table 10.8).

The tools and ideas for measures presented in this toolbox provide actors in the health care ecosystem with practical support to optimally assist those affected in the consolidation and maintenance of lifestyle changes. The tools can be used individually or in combination and coordinated between the various actors in the health care ecosystem. Their combination, coordination through different actors in the health care ecosystem as well as the possibility for personalisation support those affected in the long-term lifestyle change.

Table 10.7 Short questionnaire on motivation orientation

Question	Category	Response Scale
I personally believe that diet and exercise are important for staying healthy	Intrinsic Motivation	1 "Strongly disagree" to 5 "Strongly agree"
It is personally important to me to be healthy	Intrinsic Motivation	1 "Strongly disagree" to 5 "Strongly agree"
I do it because a professional (e.g. my doctor) said so	Extrinsic Motivation	1 "Strongly disagree" to 5 "Strongly agree"
I want others to see that I can follow my diet plan and stay fit	Extrinsic Motivation	1 "Strongly disagree" to 5 "Strongly agree"

Table 10.8 Guide to Defining Rewards

Category	Reward
Digital Reward (App)	Gamification: Badges, Status
Digital Reward (App)	Ranking (Best-in-Class-Award)
Reward through Feedback	Opportunity for Self-Monitoring
Reward through Feedback	Push-Notifications for Achievement
Real Rewards	Success-based Subsidy of Wearables
Real Rewards	Temporary Use of Sports Facilities
Real Rewards	Voucher for Personal Training
Others	Additional Challenges as Reward for Achievementss

References

Hagger, M. S., Hankonen, N. E., & Ryan, R. M. (2020). Changing behavior using self-determination theory. In M. S. Hagger, L. D. Cameron, K. Hamilton, N. Hankonen, & T. Lintunen (Eds.), *The handbook of behavior change* (S. 104–119). Cambridge University Press. https://doi.org/10.1017/9781108677318.008.

Michie, S., Richardson, M., Johnston, M., Abraham, C., Francis, J., Hardeman, W., Eccles, M. P., Cane, J., & Wood, C. E. (2013). The behavior change technique taxonomy (v1) of 93 hierarchically clustered techniques: Building an international consensus for the reporting of behavior change interventions. *Annals of Behavioral Medicine, 46*(1), 81–95. https://doi.org/10.1007/s12160-013-9486-6.

Ng, J. Y. Y., Ntoumanis, N., Thøgersen-Ntoumani, C., Deci, E. L., Ryan, R. M., Duda, J. L., & Williams, G. C. (2012). Self-determination theory applied to health contexts: A meta-analysis. *Perspectives on Psychological Science, 7*(4), 325–340. https://doi.org/10.1177/1745691612447309.